The Neurobiology of Cocaine Addiction: From Bench to Bedside

The Neurobiology of Cocaine Addiction: From Bench to Bedside

Herman Joseph, PhD
Guest Editor

Barry Stimmel, MD
Editor

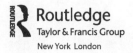

Routledge
Taylor & Francis Group
New York London

First published 1996
The Haworth Medical Press

Published 2013 by Routledge
52 Vanderbilt Avenue, New York, NY 10017
2 Park Square, Milton Park, Abingdon, Oxon OX14 4RN

Routledge is an imprint of the Taylor & Francis Group, an informa business

The Neurobiology of Cocaine Addiction: From Bench to Bedside has also been published as
Journal of Addictive Diseases, Volume 15, Number 4 1996.

Library of Congress Cataloging-in-Publication Data

The neurobiology of cocaine addiction : from bench to bedside / Herman Joseph, guest editor; Barry
Stimmel, editor.
        p. cm.–(Journal of addictive diseases ; v. 15, no. 4)
        "Has also been published as Journal of addictive diseases, volume 15, number 4,
1996"–T.p. verso.
        Includes bibliographical references and index.
        1. Cocaine habit–Physiological aspects. 2. Brain–Effect of drugs on. 3. Cocaine habit–Epi-
demiology. I. Joseph, Herman, 1931- . II. Stimmel, Barry, 1939- . III. Series.
        [DNLM: 1. Substnace Depedence–congresses. 2. Cocaine–congresses. 3. Central Nervous
System–drug effects–congresses. W1 J0533PU v. 15 no. 4 1996 / WM 280 N4943 1996]
RC568.C6N48 1996
616.86'47071–dc21
DNLM/DLC   96-39364
for Library of Congress   CIP

ISBN 13: 978-0-789-00300-3 (pbk)
ISBN 13: 978-0-789-00031-6 (hbk)

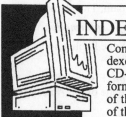# INDEXING & ABSTRACTING

Contributions to this publication are selectively in-
dexed or abstracted in print, electronic, online, or
CD-ROM version(s) of the reference tools and information services listed below. This list is current as
of the copyright date of this publication. See the end
of this section for additional notes.

- *Abstracts in Anthropology,* Baywood Publishing Company, 26 Austin
  Avenue, P.O. Box 337, Amityville, NY 11701

- *Abstracts of Research in Pastoral Care & Counseling,* Loyola
  College, 7135 Minstrel Way, Suite 101, Columbia, MD 21045

- *Academic Abstracts/CD-ROM,* EBSCO Publishing Editorial
  Department, P.O. Box 590, Ipswich, MA 01938-0590

- *ADDICTION ABSTRACTS,* National Addiction Centre, 4 Windsor
  Walk, London SE5 8AF, England

- *ALCONLINE Database,* Swedish Council for Information on Alcohol
  and Other Drugs, Box 27302, S-102 54 Stockholm, Sweden

- *Behavioral Medicine Abstracts,* University of Washington, School of
  Social Work, Seattle, WA 98195

- *Biosciences Information Service of Biological Abstracts (BIOSIS),*
  Biosciences Information Service, 2100 Arch Street, Philadelphia,
  PA 19103-1399

- *Brown University Digest of Addiction Theory and Application, The
  (DATA Newsletter),* Project Cork Institute, Dartmouth Medical
  School, 14 South Main Street, Suite 2F, Hanover, NH 03755-2015

- *Cambridge Scientific Abstracts,* Health & Safety Science Abstracts,
  Environmental Routenet (accessed via INTERNET), 7200 Wisconsin
  Avenue #601, Bethesda, MD 20814

- *Child Development Abstracts & Bibliography,* University of Kansas,
  2 Bailey Hall, Lawrence, KS 66045

- *CNPIEC Reference Guide: Chinese National Directory of Foreign
  Periodicals,* P.O. Box 88, Beijing, Peoples Republic of China

- *Criminal Justice Abstracts,* Willow Tree Press, 15 Washington Street,
  4th Floor, Newark, NJ 07102

- *Criminal Justice Periodical Index,* University Microfilms, Inc., 300
  North Zeeb Road, Ann Arbor, MI 48106

(continued)

- *Criminology, Penology and Police Science Abstracts,* Kugler Publications, P.O. Box 11188, 1001 GD Amsterdam, The Netherlands
- *Current Contents . . . .* see: *Institute for Scientific Information*
- *Educational Administration Abstracts (EAA),* Sage Publications, Inc., 2455 Teller Road, Newbury Park, CA 91320
- *Excerpta Medica/Secondary Publishing Division,* Elsevier Science Inc., Secondary Publishing Division, 655 Avenue of the Americas, New York, NY 10010
- *Family Studies Database (online and CD/ROM),* National Information Services Corporation, 306 East Baltimore Pike, 2nd Floor, Media, PA 19063
- *Health Source: Indexing & Abstracting of 160 selected health related journals, updated monthly,* EBSCO Publishing, 83 Pine Street, Peabody, MA 01960
- *Health Source Plus: expanded version of "Health Source" to be released shortly:* EBSCO Publishing, 83 Pine Street, Peabody, MA 01960
- *Index Medicus,* National Library of Medicine, 8600 Rockville Pike, Bethesda, MD 20894
- *Index to Periodical Articles Related to Law,* University of Texas, 727 East 26th Street, Austin, TX 78705
- *Institute for Scientific Information,* 3501 Market Street, Philadelphia, Pennsylvania 19104. Coverage in:
  a) Social Science Citation Index (SSCI): print, online, CD-ROM
  b) Research Alerts (current awareness service)
  c) Social SciSearch (magnetic tape)
  d) Current Contents/Social & Behavioral Sciences (weekly current awareness service)
- *International Pharmaceutical Abstracts,* ASHP, 7272 Wisconsin Avenue, Bethesda, MD 20814
- *INTERNET ACCESS (& additional networks) Bulletin Board for Libraries ("BUBL"), coverage of information resources on INTERNET, JANET, and other networks.*
  - JANET X.29: UK.AC.BATH.BUBL or 00006012101300
  - TELNET: BUBL.BATH.AC.UK or 138.38.32.45 login 'bubl'
  - Gopher: BUBL.BATH.AC.UK (138.32.32.45). Port 7070
  - World Wide Web: http: / / www.bubl.bath.ac.uk./BUBL/ home.html
  - NISSWAIS: telnetniss.ac.uk (for the NISS gateway)
  The Andersonian Library, Curran Building, 101 St. James Road, Glasgow G4 ONS, Scotland
- *Medication Use STudies (MUST) Database,* The University of Mississippi, School of Pharmacy, University, MS 38677

(continued)

- ***Mental Health Abstracts (online through DIALOG),*** IFI/Plenum Data Company, 3202 Kirkwood Highway, Wilmington, DE 19808

- ***NIAAA Alcohol and Alcohol Problems Science Database (ETOH),*** National Institute on Alcohol Abuse and Alcoholism, 1400 Eye Street NW, Suite 600, Washington, DC 20005

- ***PASCAL International Bibliography T205: Sciences de l'information Documentation,*** INIST/CNRS-Service Gestion des Documents Primaires, 2 allee du Parc de Brabois, F-54514 Vandoeuvre-les-Nancy, Cedex, France

- ***Psychological Abstracts (PsycINFO),*** American Psychological Association, P.O. Box 91600, Washington, DC 20090-1600

- ***Sage Family Studies Abstracts (SFSA),*** Sage Publications, Inc., 2455 Teller Road, Newbury Park, CA 91320

- ***Sage Urban Studies Abstracts (SUSA),*** Sage Publications, Inc., 2455 Teller Road, Newbury Park, CA 91320

- ***Social Planning/Policy & Development Abstracts (SOPODA),*** Sociological Abstracts, Inc., P.O. Box 22206, San Diego, CA 92192-0206

- ***Social Work Abstracts,*** National Association of Social Workers, 750 First Street NW, 8th Floor, Washington, DC 20002

- ***Sociological Abstracts (SA),*** Sociological Abstracts, Inc., P.O. Box 22206, San Diego, CA 92192-0206

- ***SOMED (social medicine) Database,*** Landes Institut fur Den Offentlichen Gesundheitsdienst NRW, Postfach 20 10 12, D-33548 Bielefeld, Germany

- ***Studies on Women Abstracts,*** Carfax Publishing Company, P.O. Box 25, Abingdon, Oxfordshire, OX14 3UE, United Kingdom

- ***Violence and Abuse Abstracts: A Review of Current Literature on Interpersonal Violence (VAA),*** Sage Publications, Inc., 2455 Teller Road, Newbury Park, CA 91320

(continued)

SPECIAL BIBLIOGRAPHIC NOTES

related to special journal issues (separates)
and indexing/abstracting

☐ indexing/abstracting services in this list will also cover material in any "separate" that is co-published simultaneously with Haworth's special thematic journal issue or DocuSerial. Indexing/abstracting usually covers material at the article/chapter level.

☐ monographic co-editions are intended for either non-subscribers or libraries which intend to purchase a second copy for their circulating collections.

☐ monographic co-editions are reported to all jobbers/wholesalers/approval plans. The source journal is listed as the "series" to assist the prevention of duplicate purchasing in the same manner utilized for books-in-series.

☐ to facilitate user/access services all indexing/abstracting services are encouraged to utilize the co-indexing entry note indicated at the bottom of the first page of each article/chapter/contribution.

☐ this is intended to assist a library user of any reference tool (whether print, electronic, online, or CD-ROM) to locate the monographic version if the library has purchased this version but not a subscription to the source journal.

☐ individual articles/chapters in any Haworth publication are also available through the Haworth Document Delivery Services (HDDS).

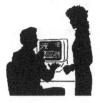

The Neurobiology of Cocaine Addiction: From Bench to Bedside

CONTENTS

ABOUT THE GUEST EDITOR

Dr. Herman Joseph is a research sociologist employed with the New York State Office of Alcoholism and Substance Abuse Services. He also holds an adjunct appointment at The Rockefeller University. As a recipient of an Aaron Diamond grant, Dr. Joseph organized the Chemical Dependency Research Working Group (CDRWG). Within the past five years the CDRWG sponsored symposia and organized projects on research and clinical issues concerning the neurobiology, epidemiology and treatment of chemical dependency; chemically dependent pregnant women and drug exposed neonates; pain management and chemical dependency; the transmission of infectious disease such as HIV; and the interrelationship of these issues with social conditions in the inner city. At The Rockefeller University, he worked with Dr. Vincent Dole and Dr. Marie Nyswander on follow-up studies of methadone maintenance patients. Dr. Joseph is co-author with Dr. David Courtwright and Dr. Don DesJarlais of the oral history, *Addicts Who Survived*. He has been an investigator on several research projects and is also the author and co-author of articles pertaining to addiction, methadone maintenance treatment, the HIV/AIDS epidemic, homelessness and the criminal justice system.

EDITORIAL

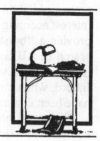

Basic Science, Epidemiology, Clinical Practice, and Philanthropy

This collection contains several papers describing patterns of cocaine use as well as the basic research that is being done in an attempt to define the reasons this drug is so reinforcing. Laboratory animals, once addicted, choose it over food and water, and in the "human laboratory" of the street, those who have become addicted also continue to take the drug despite attempts at therapy.

The selection of these papers, however, was not by chance but rather by a focused effort to bring clinicians and basic researchers together to share knowledge. Many comprise part of a symposium made possible by The Aaron Diamond Foundation's support of the Chemical Dependency Research Working Group of the New York State Office of Alcoholism and

The Chemical Dependency Research Working Group of the New York State Office of Alcoholism and Substance Abuse Services is supported by an Aaron Diamond grant to the Medical and Health Research Association of New York City, Inc.

[Haworth co-indexing entry note]: "Basic Science, Epidemiology, Clinical Practice, and Philanthropy." Joseph, Herman, and Barry Stimmel. Co-published simultaneously in *Journal of Addictive Diseases* (The Haworth Medical Press, an imprint of The Haworth Press, Inc.) Vol. 15, No. 4, 1996, pp. xv-xviii; and: *The Neurobiology of Cocaine Addiction: From Bench to Bedside* (ed: Herman Joseph, and Barry Stimmel) The Haworth Medical Press, an imprint of The Haworth Press, Inc., 1996, pp. xiii-xvi. Single or multiple copies of this article are available for a fee from The Haworth Document Delivery Service [1-800-342-9678, 9:00 a.m. - 5:00 p.m. (EST). E-mail address: getinfo@haworth.com].

Substance Abuse Services. The Aaron Diamond Foundation is unique among philanthropic organizations. Rather than providing funding from interest accruing to its endowment, the Foundation's objective has been to provide a "burst" of such great intensity into strengthening medical research in AIDS and substance abuse, by committing both principal and income for ten years, that the Foundation itself would become "extinct." Indeed, when this occurs in December 1996, more than $163 million will have been committed to support fellowships, research, and conferences.

The social and medical effects of cocaine addiction have long been known and, unfortunately, generally refractory to intervention. Frank and Galea[1] document a dramatic increase in cocaine activity, usually associated with crack, which has occurred in New York City over the past decade. Despite periods of decline, crack use has started once again to increase and has been responsible for more adverse consequences than any other illicit drug in New York City over the last ten years. It is suggested that this increase in crack use may well be related to the associated surge in heroin activity that has also been observed. Palij et al.[2] review the factors that predict daily cocaine use among patients in a methadone maintenance program. Most interesting is their observation that despite the almost irresistible craving for cocaine, time in treatment in methadone maintenance appears to be a robust predictor of reduced use. This controlled study confirms the observations of Borg et al., who found cocaine use to diminish from highs of 80% to below 20% of those remaining in methadone maintenance.[3]

Advances in the neurosciences over the past decade have emphasized the role of biological factors in the development of dependence, tolerance, and drug craving, which sustains addictive behavior. The effects of many mood-altering drugs on the pleasure/reward system of the brain result in new instinctual needs that rival the inherent instinctual drives of hunger and sex. These drug-induced biological drives are then met within the social contexts that shape human behavior. The compulsive nature of this behavior to satisfy craving has resulted in a variety of serious social and public health problems, including infectious diseases, drug-related crime, premature deaths, and community violence. Although methadone maintenance has proven an effective medical approach to treating the specific "craving" seen in heroin addiction, at present a comparable therapy does not exist for either powder cocaine or crack. However, the very nature of this dependency is currently being unraveled through neurosciences. The remaining papers in this collection review current research findings and their relevance to the clinical treatment of cocaine dependency.

It has long been known that cocaine affects the neurotransmitters, dopamine, serotonin, and norepinephrine at the neuronal levels. Prichep and colleagues[4] review studies demonstrating that persons previously dependent on cocaine displayed persistent changes in brain function not only shortly after the last crack/cocaine use but also at six months and longer. Most interesting, similar studies performed in school age children exposed in utero to crack cocaine revealed similar quantitative electrophysiological changes. These changes are believed related to dopaminergic function and increased firing of the noradrenergic cells in the locus coeruleus of the brain, with differing changes in those cocaine users who remain in treatment for more than five months, as compared to those who leave treatment earlier.

Volkow and colleagues,[5] viewing cocaine addiction through positron emission tomography (PET), describe how cocaine's affinity for the dopamine neuron is enhanced through its extremely rapid uptake in clearance from the brain. It is postulated that this rapid uptake and clearance helps explain the addictive qualities of the drug due to the intense desire for reinforcement by the cocaine user, accompanied by a loss of control.

Kreek[6] completes the circle of cocaine and heroin use by demonstrating that chronic cocaine administration not only affects those neurons concerned with dopamine, serotonin, and norepinephrine but, in addition, profoundly disrupts the endogenous opioid system. Utilizing a "binge" pattern cocaine administration model, profound dysfunction of both the dynorphine and the kappa opioid receptor genes has been demonstrated, which may facilitate the persistence of cocaine addiction. These findings may lead to another therapeutic approach utilizing drugs directed to the kappa opioid receptor to diminish or interfere with the positive reinforcement effect of cocaine. Kreek's observations may clinically explain the coexistence of cocaine and heroin addiction, the decreasing incidence of cocaine use in former heroin addicts remaining in methadone treatment, and the ability of opioids to decrease self-administration of cocaine in animal models.

Finally, Levin et al.[7] return us to the "street" by reviewing the pattern of cocaine use in those methadone-maintained persons specifically seeking entry into a study involving cocaine use. Their findings, which differ from others[8] concerning cocaine use in persons on methadone maintenance, emphasize the importance of prospective, rather than retrospective, data analysis and the limitations of a self-selective, compared to a randomized, study group. Nonetheless, their finding of a subset of heavy, consistent users of cocaine highlights the importance of seeking out more effective forms of therapy.

The papers in this collection help us understand not only the basic actions of cocaine but, equally important, the potential mechanisms that exist to alter behavior. Equally important, the funding of such seminars to allow basic scientists, epidemiologists, and clinicians to share the knowledge generated in each of their fields fosters a comprehensive understanding from the molecular to the clinical behavior seen "on the street," thereby greatly increasing the potential to diminish the craving for this drug as well as enhancing the chances of remaining abstinent.

Herman Joseph, PhD
Barry Stimmel, MD

REFERENCES

1. Frank B, Galea J. Cocaine trends and other drug trends in New York City, 1986-1994. J Addict Dis. 1996;15(4): 1-12.

2. Palij M, Rosenblum A, Magura S, Handelsman L, Stimmel, B. Daily cocaine use patterns: effects of contextual and psychological variables. J Addict Dis. 1996;15(4): 13-37.

3. Borg L, Broe DM, Ho A et al. Cocaine abuse is decreased with effective methadone maintenance treatment at an urban Department of Veterans Affairs (DVA) program. In: Harris LS, ed. Proceedings of the 56th Annual Scientific Meeting, The College on Problems of Drug Dependence, Inc., Palm Beach, Florida, June 1994. NIDA Research Monograph Series, Problems of Drug Dependence. Rockville, MD: NIH Publication No. 953883, 1995;153:17.

4. Prichep LS, Alper K, Kowalik SC, Rosenthal M. Neurometric QEEG studies of crack cocaine dependence and treatment outcome. J Addict Dis. 1996; 15(4): 39-53.

5. Volkow ND, Ding Y, Fowler JS, Wang G. Cocaine addiction: hypothesis derived from imaging studies with PET. J Addict Dis. 1996;15(4): 55-71.

6. Kreek MJ. Cocaine, dopamine and the endogenous opioid system. J Addict Dis. 1996;15(4): 73-96

7. Levin FR, Foltin RW, Fischman MW. Pattern of cocaine use in methadone maintained individuals applying for research studies. J Addict Dis. 1996;15(4): 97-106.

8. Kidorf M, Sitzer ML. Descriptive analysis of cocaine use of methadone patients. Drug Alcohol Dependence. 1993; 32:267-75.

Cocaine Trends and Other Drug Trends in New York City, 1986-1994

Blanche Frank, PhD
John Galea, MA

SUMMARY. Cocaine, mainly in the form of crack, continues to dominate New York City's illicit drug scene. Trends in cocaine-involved deaths, hospital emergencies, arrests and treatment admissions are reviewed from the late 1980s to the early 1990s. Also, street studies conducted at drug copping areas throughout New York City during this period yield ethnographic insights.

At the same time that cocaine trends were showing increases in the 1990s, heroin trends and marijuana trends were also showing decisive increases. An upsurge in heroin activity may be directly related to cocaine activity. Heroin's ameliorative effects for the cocaine user are the most direct association. The sequence–first cocaine, then heroin–has been documented by historians in the field. The association between cocaine trends and marijuana trends is less direct, and may represent the substitution of or a retreat to marijuana, a drug that is perceived as much safer. *[Article copies available for a fee from The Haworth Document Delivery Service: 1-800-342-9678. E-mail address: getinfo@ haworth.com]*

Over the past decade, New York City has seen a dramatic escalation in cocaine activity, especially associated with crack. In an effort to monitor

Blanche Frank and John Galea are affiliated with the New York State Office of Alcoholism and Substance Abuse Services, New York, NY.

[Haworth co-indexing entry note]: "Cocaine Trends and Other Drug Trends in New York City, 1986-1994." Frank, Blanche, and John Galea. Co-published simultaneously in *Journal of Addictive Diseases* (The Haworth Medical Press, an imprint of The Haworth Press, Inc.) Vol. 15, No. 4, 1996, pp. 1-12; and: *The Neurobiology of Cocaine Addiction: From Bench to Bedside* (ed: Herman Joseph, and Barry Stimmel) The Haworth Medical Press, an imprint of The Haworth Press, Inc., 1996, pp. 1-12. Single or multiple copies of this article are available for a fee from The Haworth Document Delivery Service [1-800-342-9678, 9:00 a.m. - 5:00 p.m. (EST). E-mail address: getinfo@haworth.com].

the trends, the Bureau of Applied Studies of the New York State Office of Alcoholism and Substance Abuse Services tracks a variety of drug-related indirect indicators and maintains a Street Studies Unit that observes drug activity on the streets of New York City. These information sources reveal that cocaine activity continues at high levels. At the same time, however, trends in heroin activity and in marijuana activity are also showing increases. There is evidence that these trends may be interrelated, and that the dramatic increase in cocaine activity may have contributed to an upsurge in other illicit drug activity. Given the fact that New York City, with its population of 7.3 million is the largest city in the country, has a correspondingly large drug-using subpopulation, and is also a major center of drug trafficking, New York City's drug-related trends have significance far beyond its boundaries.

INFORMATION SOURCES

This analysis draws heavily on the following indirect indicators: drug-related deaths and hospital emergency department episodes collected by the Federal Drug Abuse Warning Network (DAWN); drug-involved arrests reported by the New York City Police Department (NYPD); and treatment admissions reported by the New York State Office of Alcoholism and Substance Abuse Services (OASAS). Although each of these indicators has strengths and weaknesses in accurately reflecting drug activity, taken together they can reveal much about the drug abuse problem and the direction of specific drug trends. Deaths and hospital emergency department episodes tend to be early warning or "leading" indicators; arrests tend to follow these early warning indicators closely in time; and treatment admissions tend to be late or "lagging" indicators. Also, these indicator data have been collected in a consistent way for relatively long periods of time.

In addition, this analysis uses ethnographic findings gathered by the Street Studies Unit of the OASAS Bureau of Applied Studies. This Unit includes five men and women, who are White, Black, and Hispanic, and who are familiar with the illicit drug scene on New York City streets. In addition, they have been trained in the ethnographic gathering of information through observation and conversation with drug dealers, users and loiterers at drug copping areas and other public places throughout New York City.

COCAINE TRENDS

Table 1 presents the number of cocaine-involved deaths from 1988 through 1993, hospital emergency department episodes from 1988 through

TABLE 1. New York City Cocaine Trends for Selected Indicator Data 1986-1994

Year	Deaths Involving Cocaine[a]	Cocaine Emergency Department Mentions[b]	Cocaine Arrests[c]	State-Funded Treatment Admissions: Cocaine as Primary Drug of Abuse[d]
1986	--	--	28,594	8,140
1987	--	--	37,624	10,338
1988	1,318	16,917	49,014	10,846
1989	1,141	14,925	53,915	11,286
1990	857	12,633	46,348	11,108
1991	804	16,100	37,769	12,631
1992	730	20,413	33,708	13,072
1993	815	20,920	31,296	12,357
1994	--	19,854*	38,200	12,216

*Preliminary estimates

SOURCES: [a] SAMHSA, Drug Abuse Warning Network (DAWN) including New York City, Long Island, and Putnam County.

[b] DAWN, weighted data, based on a representative sample of hospitals for New York City, and Westchester, Rockland, and Putnam Counties.

[c] New York City Police Department.

[d] State-funded programs receive some or all funding through New York State Office of Alcoholism and Substance Abuse Services (OASAS).

1994, and arrests and treatment admissions from 1986 through 1994. Although mode of cocaine use is not specified in Table 1, crack or the "smoking" of cocaine is driving the trends. For instance, more than 80 percent of cocaine-involved arrests consistently involve crack, and more than 70 percent of treatment admissions with cocaine as the primary drug of abuse consistently report "smoking" or the use of crack as the route of administration.[1,2]

During the period of interest, from about 1986 through 1994, cocaine activity tended to peak early, decline and then increase once again:

- between 1988 and 1992 deaths involving cocaine (i.e., a "leading" indicator) declined 45 percent (from a peak of 1,318 deaths to 730 deaths), and showed a small increase of 12 percent in 1993 (815 deaths);
- between 1988 and 1990 hospital emergency episodes involving cocaine (i.e., a "leading" indicator) declined 25 percent (from a peak

of 16,917 emergencies to 12,633 emergencies); increased 66 percent between 1990 to 1993 to a second peak (20,920 emergencies);

- between 1986 and 1989, arrests involving cocaine rose 89 percent (from 28,594 arrests to 53,915 arrests), then declined 42 percent between 1989 and 1993 (from 53,915 arrests to 31,296 arrests), and increased a dramatic 22 percent in 1994 (38,200 arrests); and
- between 1986 and 1992 admissions to treatment with cocaine as the primary drug of abuse (i.e., a "lagging" indicator) rose 61 percent (from 8,140 admissions to 13,072 admissions), and declined a slight 7 percent between 1992 and 1994 (from 13,072 admissions to 12,216 admissions).

Cocaine–mainly in the form of crack–has accounted for more drug-related consequences than any other illicit drug in New York City over the past decade. Despite past evidence of declines, cocaine trends show increases once again in the most recent years.

Trends in demographic characteristics of cocaine abusers have generally remained stable. Characteristics drawn from emergency room admissions and treatment admissions tend to show that blacks represent the majority of those seeking help; that the majority of cocaine abusers are between the ages of 26 and 35 years; and that females represent about 40 percent of admissions which is the highest proportion for females in New York City for any specific illicit drug.[2]

Street Findings

For the past decade, cocaine trends were largely driven by activity surrounding crack. In the summer of 1985, the OASAS Street Studies Unit was aware of the emergence of crack in a few neighborhoods of New York City. The process by which cocaine HCl was transformed to a smokable form now used baking soda rather than a more complicated process using ether. Members of the Unit were told that the term "crack" came about because of the crackling sound the cocaine made during the heating transformation process.

Although some users prepared crack themselves, the marketing of ready-made crack on the streets quickly dominated illicit drug marketing. Small plastic vials in various sizes containing crystals of crack were sold for a range of prices from $1 to $20, depending on size. With the growing market came a large number of sellers, competing for copping locations. Given the profits to be made, dealers were vying for turf. Whether dealers were using or not, erratic and volatile behavior often characterized the marketing of crack.

Early on, the crack scene developed its own subculture, with its own language, different styles of crack pipes and other accoutrements, and crack houses where use took place and contacts were made. It was clear that addiction was occurring quickly for many users, with many running out of money. Crack-for-sex became a practice engaged in by female users and sometimes by male users, often performed in crack houses. Over the course of the decade, crack addicts–or "crack heads"–grew in number and were regarded with disgust, even among other drug users. Residents of neighborhoods where crack activity took place frequently reacted to the activity on their streets. Area residents mounted campaigns, pressured politicians and police, and often took matters into their own hands. The crack trade moved from area to area, and crack addicts were shunned all over. Nevertheless, crack continues to be the major drug marketed in New York City.

OTHER DRUG TRENDS: HEROIN AND MARIJUANA

Historically, a vast variety of illicit drugs and psychoactive prescription drugs have been sold on the streets of New York City. The specific drugs, however, that account for the most consequences (i.e., deaths, emergency room episodes, arrests and treatment admissions) in New York City remain cocaine, heroin and marijuana. In fact, 90 percent or more of New York City's drug arrests and admissions to drug abuse treatment programs involve cocaine, heroin and marijuana; more than half of drug-related deaths and drug-related hospital emergencies involve a combination of two or more of these drugs. Our focus, therefore, on other drugs will concern heroin and marijuana and their relationship to cocaine trends.[1,3,4]

Heroin Trends

Heroin has been an illicit drug of particular concern in the long term as well as in very recent years. More than 35,000 heroin addicts are in treatment at any one time in New York City. Of the 75,000 reported cases of AIDS by 1994, 46 percent involve injecting drug users; most use heroin.[5] Although heroin trends show cycles of increases and decreases over the past 25 years or more, current trends show a cycle that is increasing.

Table 2 presents heroin trend data over the past several years for four heroin-involved indirect indicators of interest: deaths, emergency department episodes, arrests and treatment admissions. In general, these indicators show sharply increasing trends in the most recent years:

- between 1990 and 1993, deaths involving heroin increased 42 percent (from 557 to 793);
- between 1990 and 1994, heroin-involved hospital emergencies almost tripled (from 3,810 to 10,892);
- after some increases and decreases between 1986 and 1994 arrests involving heroin almost doubled over this 8-year time period (from 17,289 to 33,206); and
- between 1989 and 1994, treatment admissions with heroin as the primary drug of abuse increased 27 percent (from 10,660 to 13,535).

Heroin trends had been lagging behind cocaine trends, but are most recently showing an upsurge very similar to cocaine trends.

Another indicator of importance in understanding the trends in heroin activity is the purity of street-level heroin. The Federal Drug Enforcement Administration monitors street purity over time. In the late 1980s heroin

TABLE 2. New York City Heroin Trends for Selected Indicator Data 1986-1994

Year	Deaths Involving Heroin[a]	Heroin/Morphine Emergency Department Mentions[b]	Heroin Arrests[c]	State-Funded Treatment Admissions: Heroin as Primary Drug of Abuse[d]
1986	--	--	17,289	11,223
1987	--	--	22,168	11,929
1988	833	5,394	25,152	12,246
1989	762	5,437	28,083	10,660
1990	557	3,810	24,421	11,919
1991	582	6,018	23,622	11,712
1992	679	8,382	23,509	12,569
1993	793	11,268	24,595	12,936
1994	--	10,892*	33,206	13,535

*Preliminary estimates

SOURCES: [a] SAMHSA, Drug Abuse Warning Network (DAWN) including New York City, Long Island, and Putnam County.

[b] DAWN, weighted data, based on a representative sample of hospitals for New York City, and Westchester, Rockland, and Putnam Counties.

[c] New York City Police Department.

[d] State funded programs receive some or all funding through New York State Office of Alcoholism and Substance Abuse Services.

purities in New York City tended to average below 40 percent. In the 1990s, purities have been averaging above 60 percent.[6] Given the potency of street heroin, many users were not injecting, but were sniffing or snorting heroin, and were becoming addicted. Change was taking place very rapidly. In 1988, 71 percent of primary heroin admissions to treatment reported injecting as their mode of use and 28 percent reported intranasal use; by 1994, 44 percent reported injecting and 54 percent reported intranasal use.

The trend in demographic characteristics drawn from heroin-involved hospital emergency room admissions indicate that the majority of heroin users are male, are 35 years of age or older, and are mainly Black or Hispanic. This trend generally holds true for treatment admissions with heroin as the primary drug of abuse except that Hispanics tend to be the modal group among primary heroin admissions.[2]

Also, those who report sniffing or snorting heroin as their mode of use among treatment admissions as opposed to injecting are more likely to be female, to be younger, and less likely to be white. Irrespective of mode of use, if a secondary drug of abuse is reported by primary heroin users to treatment, it is likely to be cocaine.

Heroin Street Findings

Over the past decade, the Street Studies Unit has observed the availability and use of substances on the streets of New York City, including a variety of hallucinogens, inhalants and psychoactive prescriptions drugs. The drugs, however, most sought after and sold at more copping locations are cocaine (both crack and cocaine HCl), heroin and marijuana. In recent years, however, heroin activity had declined.

Given the fact that heroin use had been tantamount to injecting drug use, and that AIDS was contracted through the shared use of unsterilized needles and associated paraphernalia, heroin had lost appeal in the late 1980s. With the availability of high purity heroin that could be sniffed or snorted instead of injected, renewed interest in heroin was taking place in the 1990s.

In conversation with drug users, the Street Studies Unit was finding that heroin served cocaine users well. First, heroin ameliorated the stimulant effects of cocaine use–especially crack use. After days of sleeplessness and hyperactivity the soothing effects of heroin were very much appreciated. Second, the "speedball" combination of heroin and cocaine–especially for the injectors–continued to be the preferred "high," touted by the most experienced users.

Currently, heroin is widely available throughout the City. Although the dime-bag or $10 bag is most available, $5 bags are also becoming more available. A variety of ethnic groups are represented among the vendors; many, however, appear to be naive and inexperienced in the drug trade.

Heroin users found at copping locations tend to be in their 30s or older. Sniffing heroin has become a vogue, with some users blatantly using on the streets and tossing away the empty glassine bags. According to the Street Studies Unit, shooting galleries may be increasing in number, which surely suggests that injecting is also increasing. A "focus group" conducted among heroin users by the Street Studies Unit elicited the conclusion from the group that despite the growing popularity of "sniffing" as the mode of heroin use, the likelihood is that injecting will eventually be the mode of use for most heroin addicts once tolerance builds and their economic resources become scarce.[7]

Marijuana Trends

Marijuana is probably the illicit drug most widely used. Although indications or consequences of use are not nearly as numerous as those involving cocaine or heroin, the trends involving marijuana are dramatically increasing after a period of decline. The marijuana-related indicator data–including hospital emergencies, arrests and treatment admissions–presented in Table 3 show the upsurge starting from about 1990 or 1991 through 1994:*

- between 1991 and 1994, hospital emergencies involving marijuana more than doubled (from 1,196 to 2,573);
- between 1991 and 1994, arrests involving marijuana increased 85 percent (from 4,762 to 8,815); and
- between 1990 and 1994 treatment admissions with marijuana as the primary drug of abuse almost doubled (from 1,662 to 3,294).

Marijuana trends are similar to heroin trends as both follow cocaine trends.

The trend in demographic characteristics of marijuana admissions to treatment indicate that they are among the youngest admissions to treatment–more than half are younger than 21 years of age. Also, more than half are Black, and three quarters are male. The vast majority are new admissions to treatment. Their secondary drug of abuse is likely to be alcohol.

---

*Deaths directly related to marijuana use are excluded because of the small number.

TABLE 3. New York City Marijuana Trends for Selected Indicator Data 1986-1994

Year	Marijuana Emergency Department Mentions[a]	Cannabis Arrests[b]	State-Funded Treatment Admissions: Marijuana as Primary Drug of Abuse[c]
1986	--	12,614	1,965
1987	--	11,457	2,155
1988	1,897	8,940	1,993
1989	1,726	7,069	1,777
1990	1,282	5,429	1,662
1991	1,196	4,762	1,737
1992	2,004	5,078	2,077
1993	2,068	6,145	2,524
1994	2,573*	8,815	3,294

*Preliminary estimates,

SOURCES: [a] SAMHSA, Drug Abuse Warning Network (DAWN) weighted data, based on a representative sample of hospitals for New York City and Westchester, Rockland, and Putnam Counties.

[b] New York City Police Department.

[c] State-funded programs receive some or all funding through New York State Office of Alcoholism and Substance Abuse Services (OASAS).

Marijuana Street Findings

Marijuana has been readily available at numerous copping locations throughout New York City. Also, numerous varieties of marijuana are available with prices that range from $100 to $500 per ounce. Their exotic brand names include "Thai Weed," "Buddha," and "Indica."

Some courier services have been discovered by the Street Studies Unit that take orders and deliver marijuana by brand right to the consumer.

Another facet of marijuana consumption concerns teenagers and young adults who have developed their unique style of marijuana use. In addition to T-shirts and caps that feature the cannabis leaf, small cigars, known as "blunts," have become a medium for use. Much of the tobacco from the cigar is removed and then replaced by marijuana and then smoked. The Street Studies Unit found this mode among inner City youth, who often combine beer drinking with their marijuana use. In a street study conducted among youth by the Unit, the sentiment expressed by some teenagers was that they were not using crack, "so who should have a problem with pot and beer?"[8]

DISCUSSION

Drug trends over the past several years in New York City indicate continued dominance of cocaine—especially in the form of crack. Since the beginning of the 1990s, however, heroin trends and marijuana trends have also been showing decisive increases. The case can be made for the direct and indirect association of these trends.

An upsurge in heroin activity after several years of significant cocaine activity is not surprising, especially in New York City, where heroin has historically been a prominent drug. This sequence in trends—first cocaine, then heroin—has been documented by historians, and has been observed in the United States as early as the 1880s, "the first cocaine epidemic."[9] It is the ameliorative effects of heroin for the cocaine user that are perhaps the most direct association between the drugs. This finding in OASAS street studies has been supported time and again. Also, as both cocaine users and heroin users become more experienced in patterns of use, the "speed-ball"—or the combining of heroin with cocaine in a variety of ways—is a use pattern that is likely to be practiced. It is also a dangerous pattern of use. Nationally speaking, DAWN mortality data have shown that 44 percent of cocaine-involved deaths also include heroin.[3]

The association between marijuana trends and cocaine trends, however, appears to be less direct, although marijuana is often a secondary drug of abuse among cocaine users. The connection may concern the "risky" way cocaine is perceived. The consequences of cocaine use—especially in the form of crack—are widely known through direct contact, media coverage, and education and prevention efforts among children. The reactions to the message may have relevance to marijuana use.

For many adults, there is the perception that cocaine, the once glamour drug, is too dangerous to use, especially in the form of crack. Marijuana on the other hand, is perceived as a much safer drug that provides enough of a "high" and enough of a disinhibiting effect to satisfy many. Also, the "pricey" varieties of cannabis that have become popular on the street give the substance an aura and status, perhaps reminiscent of cocaine. Furthermore, there is some evidence that marijuana is, in fact, stronger than ever, with a higher THC content.[10]

Teenagers and young adults in New York City show very low rates of cocaine use. The likelihood is that education and prevention efforts that focussed on cocaine—especially crack—as a dangerous drug delivered effective messages. Youth, however, do show increasing rates of marijuana use. Marijuana, by contrast, is perceived as a much safer drug. In any case, the subcultural trappings surrounding marijuana—the dress, the "blunt," the accompanying beer, the rap music–also make the substance appealing to youth, perhaps like the subcultural aspects of crack. The perception, as reported by the Street Studies Unit, "as long as I'm not using crack," may be contributing to the upsurge in marijuana use.

Finally, the drug scene is a polydrug environment. Although cocaine activity has had prominence for a decade or more, rarely are experienced drug users exclusive in their use. Alcohol is practically universal to all. In addition, a vast pharmacopeia of drugs come and go, but marijuana and heroin remain staples in New York City's drug scene. It is therefore, not surprising that cocaine, heroin and marijuana trends tend to eventually catch up with each other.

These trends do not bode well for the future. The upsurge in heroin activity, despite the sniffing or snorting as a preferred mode of use for many as they enter treatment, may ultimately result in an upsurge in injecting drug use with the associated risks for HIV disease. The upsurge in marijuana activity–especially with alcohol among a youthful population–may indicate a susceptibility for more substance abuse problems in the future. Although many drug abusers are entering treatment, patients with these particular problems are a challenge to the treatment field. Unfortunately, these problems occur at a time when the treatment field itself is undergoing major organizational change, and may well be diverted from the serious content of the problems at hand.

REFERENCES

1. New York City Police Dept. Statistical report: Complaints and arrests. 1994; 26-27.

2. Frank B, Galea J. Current drug use trends in New York City. In: Epidemiologic trends in drug abuse: Community epidemiology work group, June 1995. Rockville, MD: National Institute on Drug Abuse.

3. Substance Abuse and Mental Health Services Administration. Annual Medical examiner data, 1993. Rockville, MD: Office of Applied Studies.

4. Substance Abuse and Mental Health Services Administration. Annual emergency room data, 1992. Rockville, MD: Office of Applied Studies.

5. New York City Dept of Health. AIDS surveillance update, July 1995.

6. U.S. Dept of Justice. Domestic monitor program: 1992 annual summary. Washington, DC: Drug Enforcement Administration.

7. Frank B, Galea J. Current drug use trends in New York city. In: Epidemiologic trends in drug abuse: community epidemiology work group, June 1993. Rockville, MD: National Institute on Drug Abuse.

8. New York State Office of Alcoholism and Substance Abuse Services. Five-year comprehensive plan for alcoholism and substance abuse services, 1994-1999: 1995 update. 1994; 14-16.

9. Courtwright D. The first American cocaine epidemic. In: C/CRWG Newsletter, 1991: 1; 3-5.

10. National Narcotics Intelligence Consumers Committee. The NNICC report 1994: the supply of illicit drugs to the United States. Washington, DC: Drug Enforcement Administration, 1994; 55.

Daily Cocaine Use Patterns:
Effects of Contextual
and Psychological Variables

Michael Palij, PhD
Andrew Rosenblum, PhD
Stephen Magura, PhD
Leonard Handelsman, MD
Barry Stimmel, MD

SUMMARY. This study identifies factors that predict daily cocaine use among clients in a methadone maintenance program who participated in a cocaine treatment trial. Cocaine use decreased the longer clients remained in treatment, and the amount of cocaine used depended upon the day of the week, with Saturday typically having the greatest use and Sunday having the least. Logistic regression analyses showed that several other factors were related to daily cocaine use: peak cocaine craving, resistance to use cocaine, and several triggers or stimuli to use cocaine. These stimuli included receiving

Michael Palij, Andrew Rosenblum, and Stephen Magura are affiliated with the National Development and Research Institutes, Inc., New York, NY. Michael Palij is also affiliated with Yeshiva University, New York, NY.

Leonard Handelsman and Barry Stimmel are affiliated with Narcotics Rehabilitation Center and Mount Sinai Hospital, New York, NY.

Address correspondence to: Michael Palij, PhD, NDRI, Two World Trade Center, New York, NY 10048. Email: palij@xp.psych.nyu.edu

This research was supported by Grant No. 5 R18 DA06959 from the National Institute on Drug Abuse to National Development and Research Institutes, Inc.

[Haworth co-indexing entry note]: "Daily Cocaine Use Patterns: Effects of Contextual and Psychological Variables." Palij, Michael et al. Co-published simultaneously in *Journal of Addictive Diseases* (The Haworth Medical Press, an imprint of The Haworth Press, Inc.) Vol. 15, No. 4, 1996, pp. 13-37; and: *The Neurobiology of Cocaine Addiction: From Bench to Bedside* (ed: Herman Joseph, and Barry Stimmel) The Haworth Medical Press, an imprint of The Haworth Press, Inc., 1996, pp. 13-37. Single or multiple copies of this article are available for a fee from The Haworth Document Delivery Service [1-800-342-9678, 9:00 a.m. - 5:00 p.m. (EST). E-mail address: getinfo@haworth.com].

money, being offered cocaine, and seeing cocaine and/or related paraphernalia. However, even with these variables controlled, day of the week and time in treatment continued to be significant predictors. This suggests that (a) other time-varying variables need to be included in order to fully account for cocaine use variation from day to day and (b) time in treatment is a robust predictor of reduced cocaine use despite the strong influences of craving, external stimuli, and day of the week. *[Article copies available for a fee from The Haworth Document Delivery Service: 1-800-342-9678. E-mail address: getinfo@ haworth.com]*

Cocaine is a powerfully addictive substance, but this fact alone does not allow us to predict the regularity with which cocaine will be used. Numerous conditioning studies with animals have established that cocaine is a powerful reinforcer of behavior and that animals will engage in complex schedules of reinforcement to obtain cocaine.[1] One of the more important results from this work is that animals can be brought under stimulus control to obtain cocaine; that is, they will attend to changes in stimulus conditions and when a stimulus signals the availability of the drug, will begin to respond to obtain cocaine.

Childress and her associates have done significant work extending conditioning principles to human drug use.[2-5] Their studies showed that when cocaine users are exposed to cocaine related stimuli, they undergo physiological changes such as decreases in skin temperature and skin resistance, and increases in heart rate, cocaine craving, and withdrawal symptoms.[6,7] An additional interesting result is that a person's mood may also serve as a conditioned stimulus eliciting craving or withdrawal symptoms.[8,9] This means that negative mood states, such as depression or anxiety, may serve as triggers to craving, which in turn may lead to drug use.

There are several significant aspects to these results. First, the types of conditioned responses made in the laboratory also appear in clinical and real life settings, demonstrating that conditioning principles are probably influencing everyday cocaine use.[3] Second, from a behavioral treatment perspective, if cocaine use is a response to craving and withdrawal symptoms brought on by conditioned stimuli, then it should be possible to break the link between the conditioned stimuli and the conditioned responses of craving and withdrawal through the process of extinction, that is, repeated exposure to conditioned stimuli (e.g., a crack pipe) without reinforcement (i.e., smoking crack).[3,10] This latter point has clear clinical significance and Childress and her colleagues have followed through with the development of treatment procedures based on these results.[11,12]

Although the research on the role of conditioning principles shows promise both in providing greater understanding of the factors that affect and maintain cocaine use, as well as in providing clinical techniques for treating cocaine use, it may not provide a complete accounting of why cocaine use occurs. Cognitive approaches, which focus on information-processing strategies and processes have also been suggested as pertinent[13] and these approaches may provide additional insights into drug use since factors like language, beliefs, and attitudes are considered. Conditioning approaches are fundamentally oriented toward the establishment of associations between stimuli and responses, while cognitive models may make use of other mechanisms or associations to link stimuli to responses. For instance, many information processing models make use of symbolic representations of stimuli, apply rules to these symbols and then use the results of this processing as the basis for the observed response (e.g., Anderson's ACT* model[14]). From a cognitive perspective it is how the stimulus is processed and/or interpreted that serves as the focus because this should result in behavior.

In Tiffany's[13] model (which is based on the automatic processing vs. controlled processing distinction developed by Schneider & Shiffrin[15,16]), drug craving develops in response to the automatic activation of drug use schemas stored in one's memory. In the long-term drug user, the activation of the schema occurs outside of consciousness and initiates craving which leads to actual drug use. However, although this activation is automatic, it can be affected by other cognitive processes which are under conscious control, which can intervene and attempt to prevent the schema from being translated into drug use. The treatment implications are clear: identify appropriate cognitive strategies that will disrupt the automatic cognitive processing and give the person the option of preventing drug use. A variety of cognitive-behavioral approaches either explicitly or implicitly recognized the role of such cognitive processes.[17-19]

This review leads to the following conclusions:

1. Drug use may be significantly dependent upon the occurrence of specific conditioned stimulus events, either external stimuli, such as the appearance of materials or people associated with drug use, or internal stimuli, such as negative mood states.
2. Although these stimuli ultimately lead to drug use, their effects may be mediated by craving and avoidance of withdrawal.

This raises the question of whether one can identify a relatively simple model that will predict the timing of cocaine use, given relevant information about external stimuli, mood states, and degree of craving. One must also examine whether other factors need to be taken into account or whether these variables are sufficient in predicting cocaine use. We present the results of such an attempt, based on the analysis of daily cocaine use by patients in a methadone maintenance program who were also enrolled in a cocaine treatment trial. Based on patients' reports of their daily cocaine use, exposure to various stimuli, and ratings of cocaine craving and resistance, we attempt to identify a simple model that describes the variables predicting daily cocaine use.

METHOD

Patients

The data come from patients who participated in a larger research/demonstration project that was adapting and evaluating a manual-driven cognitive-behavioral based treatment for stimulant abuse[19] within an urban methadone maintenance program.[20] This project included a medication trial that examined whether the dopamine agonist bromocriptine was effective in reducing cocaine craving and/or use.[21] Patients (all male) received either bromocriptine or placebo under double-blind conditions in addition to cognitive-behavioral therapy. Thirty-nine of these 50 patients who participated in the medication study had complete data for the 42 days of the medication trial.

Patients began participation on a Monday and spent the first week in a pre-treatment phase (i.e., no medication, no cognitive-behavioral therapy), followed by a five week treatment period. Patients reported to the methadone clinic six days a week for their daily dose of methadone (which they took under supervision) and participation in the clinic's activities. The clinic is closed on Sunday; on Saturday patients were given a take home dose of methadone to be self-administered on Sunday.

Study eligibility was determined by a DSM-III-R diagnosis of cocaine dependence, at least one cocaine positive urine in the month before study entry, no psychotic disorder, and stabilized methadone dose. Patients were excluded if they had a serious medical or psychiatric condition (e.g., psychotic disorder, cardiac disease) for which bromocriptine would be contraindicated. Women were excluded from the medication trial since bromocriptine is contraindicated during pregnancy and almost all of the women at the clinical site were of child bearing potential. Participation in the study was voluntary; all patients signed an informed consent.

Table 1 provides background characteristics of the patients. Patients ranged in age from 24 to 62 years, both the mean and median age being 39

TABLE 1. Subject characteristics.

Age	*Mean*	39.30	
	Std Dev	8.90	
	N	39	
Number of Days cocaine was used in	*Mean*	18.26	
the 30 days prior to entry into study	*Std Dev*	9.06	
	N	39	
Number of Days with four or	*Mean*	1.54	
more drinks of alcohol	*Std dev*	4.88	
	(*Minimum* = 0.00, *Maximum* = 26)		
	N	39	
Months in Methadone Program	*Mean*	40.06	
	Std dev	46.21	
	N	38	
Dose of Methadone	*Mean*	75.53	
	Std dev	18.26	
	N	38	

Ethnic Group		*Frequency*	*Percent*
	Black	12	30.8
	Hispanic	21	53.8
	White	3	7.7
	Asian/Pacific Island	1	2.6
	Other	2	5.1
	Total	39	100.0

Occupational Status		*Frequency*	*Percent*
	Employed full time	2	5.1
	Employed part time	7	17.9
	Unemployed not looking	21	53.8
	Unemployed looking	9	23.1
	Total	39	100.0

Highest Grade (Educational		*Frequency*	*Percent*
Level) Completed	9th Grade	11	28.2
	10th Grade	3	7.7
	11th Grade	9	23.1
	12th Grade	5	12.8
	Some college	4	10.3
	Associate degree	4	10.3
	College degree	3	7.7
	Total	39	100.0

years. Cocaine was used a median of 20 days in the 30 days prior to entry into the study. The majority of the sample was Hispanic (54%) and African-American (31%). Twenty-three percent were employed at time of study entry. Educational achievement was varied, with 28% completing only the 9th grade but 8% reporting having a college degree. The current residence of the majority of the patients was either someone else's house or apartment (46%) or their own home or apartment (36%); 5% of the patients reported living on the street. At intake 16% were on probation, on parole, or were out on bail. The majority of patients were Christian.

Materials and Procedure

Patients were administered questionnaires on their background, current emotional status, and current activities. One of these questionnaires, the Cocaine Craving Questionnaire (CCQ), was developed on the basis of clinical judgment and knowledge of relevant factors from the research literature. Patients completed the CCQ three times a week (Monday, Wednesday, and Friday), reporting on either the previous two or three days. The CCQ elicited reports of daily medication compliance, cocaine use, cocaine craving, resistance to cocaine use, and exposure to stimuli which may lead to cocaine craving and/or use. Cocaine craving and resistance to using cocaine were rated on a 100 mm visual analog scale (i.e., patients indicated their degree of craving or resistance by making a mark on a straight line 100 mm long, with zero signifying no craving [or maximum resistance] and 100 maximum craving [or least resistance]). Patients were provided a list of 12 Stimulus-To-Use (STU) events (e.g., seeing cocaine, feeling bad) which required a Yes (occurred) or No response. They reported on the occurrence of STUs regardless of cocaine usage on any particular day.

RESULTS

This section is divided into two parts: (1) a presentation of descriptive analyses for self-reported daily cocaine use, levels of cocaine craving, levels of resistance to cocaine use, and exposure to stimuli that may elicit cocaine use, and (2) a presentation of inferential analyses that attempt to predict daily cocaine use from the craving, resistance, and exposure to STU variables.

Descriptive Analyses

Self-Reported Daily Cocaine Usage. Daily cocaine use for 42 continuous days was obtained for 39 patients from responses on the CCQ and from therapists' session notes which identified whether cocaine has been used. The 42 days of data are conceptualized as representing a two-factor within-subject or repeated measures design with *Week in Study* as one within-subject factor comprised of six levels (Pre-treatment week and five weeks in treatment) and *Day of the Week* as a second within-subject factor comprised of seven levels (Monday through Sunday). This type of design was used as the basis for a repeated measures ANOVA which will be presented later.

Patients provided information on how much cocaine they used (in dollar amounts) and the route of administration on a daily basis. For those patients who reported cocaine use on a particular day, the mean dollar amount of cocaine/crack use was $26 and the median was $20 (one subject reported spending no money; otherwise, the minimum was $2 and the maximum was $500; N = 767 days reported upon by patients). For those reporting cocaine/crack use and providing information on how it was used, the most common mode of administration was by smoking crack which was reported on 71% of the days on which cocaine was used, followed by IV coke use on 34% of the days, and sniffing of cocaine on 23% of the days (note that some patients used multiple routes of administration which explains why the sum of the percentages exceed 100%).

Table 2 provides the proportion of times cocaine was used for each day of the week with the unit of analysis being subject-days. That is, the proportion for each day of the week is based on all of the data available for that day. This produces 234 values, based on 39 patients times 6 weeks in which the day occurs (i.e., the number of times each day of the week is reported on by each subject). The proportion of cocaine use takes 234 as the denominator for the proportion and the number of days cocaine use was reported in the numerator. Thus, on Monday, cocaine was used on about 43% of the opportunities (i.e., 101 out of 234 opportunities for cocaine use). The pattern in Table 2 shows moderate cocaine use during the week, peak usage on Saturday, and lowest daily use on Sunday. The difference in cocaine use from Saturday to Sunday is quite dramatic, .32 point drop in proportion of cocaine used. Figure 1 more clearly shows this daily variation in cocaine use.

Rated Cocaine Craving and Resistance to Use Cocaine. Figure 2 provides a graphic representation of the daily variation in mean ratings for three measures: peak cocaine craving, average cocaine craving, and resistance to cocaine use. Focusing first on craving, both peak and average craving show similar day-to-day variation even though the ratings for peak cravings are about 10 mm greater in value. The range of variation is somewhat restricted when one focuses on Monday through Saturday

TABLE 2. Subject-days based proportion of cocaine use.

Group-Based Proportion	Day of Week							Row Total
	Monday	Tuesday	Wednesday	Thursday	Friday	Saturday	Sunday	
Self-Reported Cocaine Use Prop. Cocaine Used	.43	.38	.38	.38	.41	.54	.22	.39

Note: Each proportion is based on the number of reported cocaine uses divided by the total number of opportunities for cocaine use (i.e., each subject contributes 6 data points, one for each week (therefore Daily N = 39 patients × 6 weeks or 234 values; *Total N = 39 patients × 7 days of week × 6 weeks or 1638 values).

FIGURE 1. Self-reported cocaine use for each day of the week, averaged across the six weeks in the study.

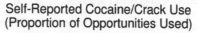

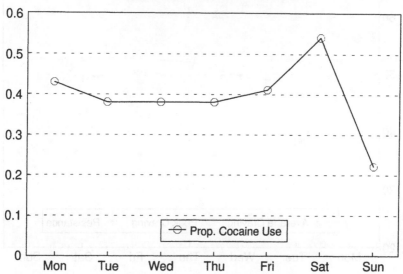

(peak: 48-53 mm; average craving: 38-44 mm), but there is a dramatic drop in craving from Saturday to Sunday (about 9-11 mm), mirroring the drop in cocaine use represented in Table 2. Resistance shows the opposite pattern. Resistance to use cocaine has limited variability from Monday to Saturday (47-54) while there is an 11 mm increase from Saturday to Sunday.

The results thus far indicate that cocaine use, cocaine craving, and resistance to using cocaine appear dependent upon the day of the week, with Saturday and Sunday having the greatest departures from fairly stable weekday levels. To explore the possibility that this variation is due to differences in daily exposure to stimuli that elicit cocaine use, the following sections focus on the subjects' reports of having been exposed to 12 different cocaine eliciting Stimulus-To-Use (STU) conditions.

Figure 3 graphically represents the daily variations for the following STU variables: having received money, being offered cocaine, and having seen cocaine or related paraphernalia. For all three variables there is a fairly stable pattern of occurrence with the largest changes occurring be-

FIGURE 2. Rated cocaine craving and resistance to use cocaine for each day of the week, averaged across the six weeks in the study.

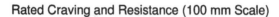

Rated Craving and Resistance (100 mm Scale)

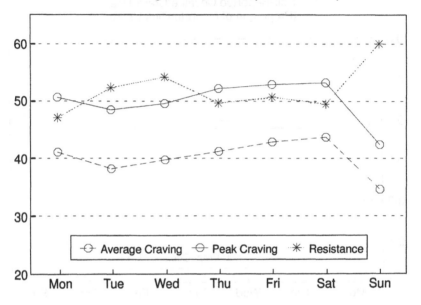

tween Saturday and Sunday. Sunday is uniformly lowest in occurrence of these variables while Saturday tends to have the highest level of occurrence. These patterns agree quite well with the results for cocaine use, craving, and resistance, suggesting an overall pattern of covariation.

Figure 4 represents the daily variation for three variables: use of alcohol or tranquilizers, having a good thing happen, and having a bad thing happen. The pattern here is somewhat different, with Sunday tending to be lowest in occurrence, though not for "having a bad thing happen," for which Friday has the least occurrence. Saturday no longer represents the day of greatest occurrence. This suggests that there is much less covariation between these variables and the previous STU variables.

Figure 5 shows the daily variation for having felt up, having felt down, and having been busy. Here that patterns tend to differ markedly from the earlier cocaine use variables, with the weekend effect either attenuated or absent altogether.

Figure 6 shows the daily variation for having been bored, having had a vivid drug dream, and having felt angry. The levels of occurrence for drug

FIGURE 3. Self-reported STU variables exposure: received money, was offered cocaine, and saw cocaine or cocaine-related paraphernalia/works for each day of the week.

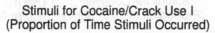

Stimuli for Cocaine/Crack Use I
(Proportion of Time Stimuli Occurred)

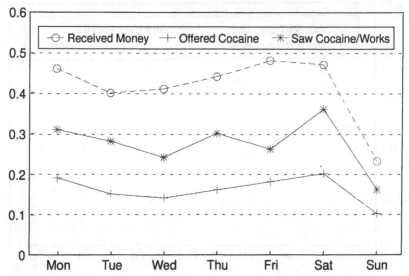

dreams and feeling angry are fairly low and remain fairly stable across the week, although there is a small tendency for feeling angry to decline over the course of the week. Being bored also shows a decline over the course of the week. None of these variables show the weekend effect and do not appear to covary with cocaine use.

Summarizing the patterns that were obtained for the stimuli that may elicit cocaine use, we see that several variables, such as receiving money, being offered cocaine, and seeing cocaine or cocaine related paraphernalia, have day-to-day variations similar to that seen for cocaine use. Most of the other STU variables had the lowest frequency of occurrence on Sunday but otherwise had a pattern that did not appear to covary with daily cocaine use.

Inferential Analyses

The inferential analyses consist of two parts: (1) an initial repeated measures ANOVA and (2) logistic regressions to confirm the ANOVA

FIGURE 4. Self-reported STU variables exposure: used alcohol or tranquilizers, had a bad thing happen, and had a good thing happen for each day of the week.

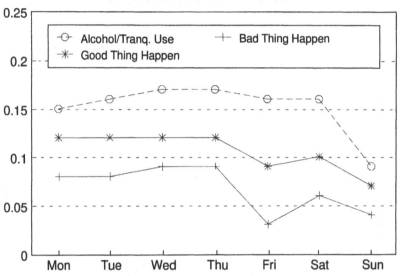

Stimuli for Cocaine/Crack Use II
(Proportion of Time Stimuli Occurred)

results and to build a prediction model that allows identification of factors predicting cocaine use. In the ANOVA analyses the *subject* served as the unit of analysis (with each subject having 42 days of data), while in the logistic regression analyses the *subject-day* served as the unit of analysis. In the ANOVA analyses, only patients with complete cocaine use data were used (N = 39). In the logistic regression analyses, although all 39 patients were included in the analyses, all 39 did not have data on all of the predictors for each day (such as craving ratings or the STU variables). In terms of subject-days (the unit of analysis used in the logistic regressions) less than 6% had missing data. All subject-days that had complete data for the variables were included in the analysis.

Repeated Measures ANOVA Results. As discussed earlier, this study can be conceptualized as a factorial design with *Week in Study* and *Day of Week* as two separate within-subject factors. This analysis also includes a dichotomous third factor, medication group, giving an active medication vs. placebo by Week in study by Day of week factorial design.

FIGURE 5. Self-reported STU variables exposure: felt down, felt up, and was busy for each day of the week.

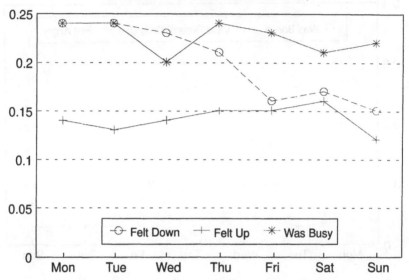

Stimuli for Cocaine/Crack Use III
(Proportion of Time Stimuli Occurred)

The first analysis that was conducted was a repeated measures ANOVA on the $2 \times 6 \times 7$ design with the dependent variable being a dichotomous variable representing either absence of cocaine use (coded zero) or reported cocaine use (coded one). The significance tests are therefore concerned with significant differences among the proportions calculated for each of the factors and their interactions. The ANOVA provided only two statistically significant results: (1) a main effect due to day of week ($F[6,222] = 10.15$, $p < .0001$) and (2) a main effect due to week in study ($F[5,185] = 7.12$, $p < .0001$). The week in study effect indicates that there is a significant decline in cocaine use from the pre-treatment week (.49) to fifth week in treatment (.30). Since this effect is independent of the day of the week effect (i.e., this is a main effect and there was no interaction between week in study and day of week), we will have no more to say about this effect here. This effect represents the efficacy of the cognitive-behavioral treatment which is reported elsewhere.[20,22]

The main effect for day of the week is represented in Table 2 and in Figure 1. The effect is most likely due to the difference between the most

FIGURE 6. Self-reported STU variables exposure: was bored, had a vivid dream about drug use, and felt angry.

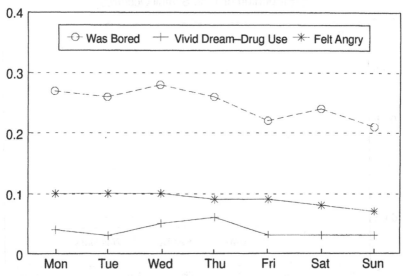

Stimuli for Cocaine/Crack Use IV
(Proportion of Time Stimuli Occurred)

extreme proportions, that is, between the most extreme cocaine use values which are on Saturday (.54) and Sunday (.22). A caveat is that although performing a repeated measures ANOVA on a dichotomous dependent variable can be justified[23] it does violate one of the assumptions required for valid ANOVA, namely, that the dependent variable (or more correctly, the errors) be normally distributed (see Aldrich & Nelson[24]). It is unclear how robust the repeated measures ANOVA is with respect to this violation or some of the other problems posed by the use of dichotomous dependent variable. There are several other methods for analyzing a dichotomous dependent variable which vary in their degree of complexity. One appropriate alternative method is to conduct a logistic regression where the dichotomous dependent variable of cocaine use is regressed on predictors such as appropriately coded design variables. We now turn to the results of such analyses.

Logistic Regression Analyses. Which variables should be used in the logistic regression analysis? Table 3 provides information on the relationship between cocaine use and the craving/resistance measures and the

TABLE 3. Relationship of craving, resistance, and STU variables to cocaine use and design factors shown to be related to cocaine use (Day as unit of analysis).

Craving, Resistance, & STU	Corr. with Cocaine Use r (N)	Day of Week	Week in Study
Peak Cocaine Craving	.53*** (1549)		
Average Cocaine Craving	.44*** (1594)		
Resistance to Cocaine Use	−.45*** (1549)		
Received Money	.40*** (1559)	***	n.s.
Offered Cocaine	.33*** (1995)	*	n.s.
Saw Cocaine/Paraphernalia	.47*** (1560)	***	***(D)
Drank Alcohol/Tranquilizer	.01 (1557)	n.s.	n.s.
Bad Thing Happened	.09*** (1558)	+	n.s.
Good Thing Happened	.04+ (1558)	n.s.	n.s.
Felt Down	.18*** (1558)	*	***(D)
Felt Up	.02 (1549)	n.s.	***(D)
Busy & Active	−.03 (1558)	n.s.	**(D)
Was Bored	.23*** (1557)	n.s.	***(D)
Vivid Drug Dream	−.0069 (1556)	n.s.	***(D)
Felt Angry	.08** (1551)	n.s.	**(D)

Note:
1. (D) = negative coefficient; n.s. = not significant
+ = .05 < p < .10
* = p < .05
** = p < .01
*** = p < .001

2. Columns titled "Day of Week" and "Week in Study" represent significance of the regression coefficients for these variables from logistic regressions in which the STU variables were regressed on these two design factors.

STU variables. The rows of Table 3 identify the craving, resistance and STU variables. The first column of numbers contains the zero-order Pearson between these variables and cocaine use (these are point-biserial coefficients for the continuous craving and resistance and phi coefficients for the dichotomous STU variables) and the number of values used in the calculation. Recall that subject-day serves as the unit of analysis here, thus every subject potentially contributes 42 pairs of values. The cocaine craving and resistance to use variables are statistically significant, but more importantly they are substantial in size, ranging from .44 to .53 in absolute value, reflecting a moderately strong relationship between cocaine use and rated craving and resistance to use.

The remainder of the first column of Table 3 contains the correlations between cocaine use and the STU variables; although the sample size is very large only a little more than half are statistically significant. The strongest relationships are between cocaine use and the three variables representing external stimuli: receiving money, being offered cocaine, and seeing cocaine or related paraphernalia. Modest correlations are seen for being bored and having felt down. Having had something bad happen and having felt angry are significantly but weakly correlated with cocaine use.

Additional analyses were conducted on the STU variables to determine whether they were related to day of the week and week in treatment (i.e., the two main effects associated with daily cocaine use). Logistic regressions using the STU variables as dependent variables and day of the week and week in study as predictors were conducted; the results are presented in the last two columns of Table 3. Only four STU variables had a significant relationship to day of the week: having received money, being offered cocaine, having seen cocaine or paraphernalia, and having felt down. Several of the STU variables are related to week in study but, oddly enough, the coefficients for all of these variables are negative, indicating that frequency of occurrence of these variables decreased as time in the study went on. For some of the STU variables this is a sensible result (e.g., saw cocaine or paraphernalia, felt down, was bored, felt angry, having a vivid drug dream) because they are explainable in terms of therapeutic effects (i.e., therapy helped the subject to avoid these situations), but it is not clear why feeling up or being busy and active would go down.

In a preliminary analysis based on a subset of patients and reported by Palij[25] and his colleagues, a logistic regression equation was obtained for daily cocaine use with the following predictors: day of week, week in study, peak cocaine craving, average cocaine craving, resistance to cocaine use, having received money, having been offered cocaine, and having seen cocaine and/or paraphernalia. The pattern of zero-order correlations shown in Table 3 is still consistent with this model, suggesting that it is a reasonable starting point. We used this model for the present data and found that average daily craving was no longer a significant predictor. It was excluded and the analysis was re-done. This model, based on the equation predicting cocaine use from day of week, week in study, peak cocaine craving, resistance to cocaine use, having received money, having been offered cocaine, and having seen cocaine and/or paraphernalia, is now examined in detail.

Table 4 provides the classification table relating the observed cocaine use status to the predicted status based on the model. This model has an overall accuracy of 88% and is somewhat better at predicting cocaine abstinence (91%) than cocaine use (83%). The fit of the model to the data was assessed by the Hosmer and Lemeshow Goodness of Fit test[26] (Chi-squared value of 8.88, df = 8, p = .35). The nonsignificant Chi-squared value indicates that there is close agreement between the values predicted by the model and observed values. On this basis, we can claim that the model, as presently constituted, acceptably predicts when cocaine use occurs.

Examination of the roles played by the different variables in the model provides additional insight into the current model. Table 5 lists the variables in the model, their regression coefficients, significance levels, and odds ratios. With respect to day of the week, overall it is a significant factor (as represented by the first line in Table 5) but the individual variables that represent the contrast between a particular day and Sunday are not all statistically significant. The coefficients representing the Thursday-Sunday and Friday-Sunday contrasts are clearly not significant while those for Monday-Sunday and Tuesday-Sunday are marginally significant (i.e., .05 < p < .10). The Wednesday-Sunday coefficient is clearly significant but the strongest effect is shown by the Saturday-Sunday coefficient which has an odds ratio of 4.3, indicating that use of cocaine on Saturday is over 4 times more likely than on Sunday.

TABLE 4. Classification table relating the observed cocaine use status to the predicted status based on the simultaneous logistic regression model.

Observed	Predicted		Percent Correct
	Abstinent	Using	
Abstinent	847	82	91.17%
Using	103	511	83.22%
		Overall	88.01

TABLE 5. Logistic regression coefficients from simultaneous model consisting of week in study, day of the week, peak craving, resistance to use, receiving money, offered cocaine, and seeing cocaine and/or paraphernalia.

Variable	B	S.E.	Wald	df	Sig	R	Exp (B)
Day of Week			25.6272	6	.0003	.0811	
Mon-Sun (1)	.5475	.3236	2.8627	1	.0907	.0204	1.7289
Tue-Sun (2)	.5590	.3272	2.9183	1	.0876	.0210	1.7489
Wed-Sun (3)	.8079	.3207	6.3461	1	.0118	.0458	2.2432
Thu-Sun (4)	.2110	.3268	.4166	1	.5186	.0000	1.2349
Fri-Sun (5)	.4690	.3307	2.0121	1	.1560	.0024	1.5985
Sat-Sun (6)	1.4590	.3279	19.7967	1	.0000	.0926	4.3016
Week in Study	−.1326	.0497	7.1093	1	.0077	−.0496	.8758
Peak Craving	.0462	.0031	225.1455	1	.0000	.3280	1.0473
Resistance	−.0408	.0030	188.4984	1	.0000	−.2998	.9600
Received Money	.8372	.1692	24.4724	1	.0000	.1041	2.3100
Offered Cocaine	.9164	.2604	12.3832	1	.0004	.0708	2.5003
Saw Cocaine	1.8821	.1969	91.3222	1	.0000	.2075	6.5672
Constant	−2.2501	.3341	45.3485	1	.0000		

Variables in the Equation

Week in Study has a negative coefficient and an odds ratio less than one, indicating that the longer patients remained in treatment, the lower the likelihood that cocaine would be used. Rated peak cocaine craving has a positive but deceptively small coefficient and an odds ratio close to one. Recall that peak cocaine craving is rated on a 100 mm scale. Thus the coefficient and the odds ratio reflect changes relative to a 1 mm change on the scale. For current purposes we are content to acknowledge that cocaine use increases as the level of peak craving increases (additional analyses which converted the continuous variables into categories were conducted but provided no real changes in interpretation). Rated resistance to cocaine use also uses the 100 mm scale but here we see a negative coefficient and an odds ratio of less than one. The simplest interpretation to be made is that as resistance increases, the likelihood of cocaine use decreases. Receiving money increases the likelihood of using cocaine, as represented by the odds ratio of 2.3. Being offered cocaine increases the likelihood of cocaine use by 2.5. Finally, seeing cocaine or paraphernalia has the biggest effect, producing an odds ratio of 6.6, meaning that a person seeing cocaine or related paraphernalia is about six and half times more likely to use cocaine than a person who does not.

Another logistic regression analysis was performed to answer the following question: would we still obtain this model if all of the STU and craving/resistance variables were allowed to enter? A forward stepwise procedure (with a Likelihood Ratio criterion for entry/deletion) was used and the current model re-emerged along with two additional variables ("having drank alcohol or taken a tranquilizer" and "indicating that one was bored"). This nine predictor model raises the overall correct prediction level to 88.33% from the 88.01% for the earlier 7 predictor model, a trivial increase. The inclusion of the two new predictors does not seem to add anything statistically or substantively to the model and makes it less parsimonious. For these reasons, it seems more appropriate to settle on the simpler seven predictor model.

In summary, a prediction model for daily cocaine use was developed and indicates the importance of cognitive-behavioral treatment (as represented by the weeks in treatment variable), day of the week (especially Saturday vs. Sunday), peak cocaine craving, perceived resistance to cocaine use, and three external triggers to cocaine use. The model appears to account for both cocaine abstinence and cocaine use, allowing prediction with a reasonable degree of accuracy of whether these patients are likely to use cocaine on any given day.

DISCUSSION

The results of the logistic regression analyses lead us to the following conclusion: the model that most parsimoniously predicts whether cocaine use will occur on any given day depends upon the following factors:

1. Day of week
2. Weeks in treatment (i.e., length of time)
3. Self-rated peak craving for cocaine
4. Self-rated resistance to use cocaine
5. Whether one received money on that particular day
6. Whether one was offered cocaine on that particular day
7. Whether one saw cocaine or related paraphernalia on that particular day.

Several of these factors, such as 3-7 above, have been previously hypothesized or observed as being related to cocaine/crack use, so their emergence here is consistent with previous research. Week in treatment is a significant factor, predicting reduction in cocaine use the longer patients stay in the cognitive-behavioral treatment program; this provides one measure of the efficacy of treatment. The question remains of why does day of the week remain a significant predictor after other obvious factors related to cocaine/crack use have been included?

Several explanations are possible, perhaps some more reasonable than others:

1. The Social Activity/Party Time-Family Time Hypothesis. The weekend may be seen as a time for social contact and having fun, hence, cocaine use should increase on Friday and Saturday as a result of its concomitant use in social activities as going to parties, clubs, and other social venues. By the same reasoning, social activities on Sunday may occur in very different circumstances (e.g., spending the day with family members who are not cocaine abusers in situations that make cocaine use difficult). The way to test for this would be to include a variable identifying the type of social activity that one is engaged in during the day, comparable to STU exposure variables, and then using this as a predictor in the model. If this were the case then two results might be produced: (a) an increase in correct prediction because the remaining factor(s) systematically related to cocaine use would be included in the model, and (b) day of the week may drop from the model *if* no other time-varying variables are involved in this situation. Unfortunately, information on social activities was not collected in any systematic fashion though anecdotally patients did report that social activities influenced cocaine use in the manner described above. Currently we are undertaking a systematic examination of daily activity patterns for a select group of patients.

It should be noted that though the Social Activity hypothesis is intuitively compelling as an explanation for explaining daily variation in cocaine use it may not be the only factor that is influencing daily use. Although social context may set the stage for cocaine use one still must ask why cocaine use would occur, that is, why does not a person simply refuse to use in social settings. Social pressures and situation factors are probably operating but the situational factors may not be only social in nature. Instead, stimuli in social situations may serve an eliciting or signalling function (i.e., they are conditioned stimuli) and require additional psychological mechanisms as explanatory devices. We identify some of these mechanisms after considering some other explanations for the Saturday-Sunday difference in cocaine use.

2. The Cocaine Hangover Hypothesis. The difference in cocaine/crack use from Saturday to Sunday could be due to a hangover effect, that is, excessive use on Saturday night incapacitates the user on Sunday, thus causing a reduction in use because the user is unable to engage in behaviors necessary to procure and use cocaine. This is an unlikely explanation because cocaine's action is not comparable to that of alcohol where hangover effects are most obvious. Although exhaustion can arise with prolonged and extreme cocaine use, it does not appear to characterize the patients in this study because they reported that they still engaged in various activities on Sunday. Moreover, though this explains why cocaine use would be reduced on Sunday, it does not explain why cocaine use is increased on Saturday.

3. *The Cocaine Satiation Hypothesis.* The reason why cocaine use may be down on Sunday is because Saturday's use satisfies all of the cocaine craving that a person may have for the immediate future. Although cocaine craving is reduced on Sunday and resistance is up on Sunday, patterns that are supportive of a cocaine satiation explanation, it is unlikely that satiation is the mechanism that is operating. From animal studies[1] and anecdotal reports from crack users, there does not appear to be a satiation point in cocaine use. Animals will continue to barpress for cocaine even though they are starving and dehydrating themselves to death. Crack users may purchase hundreds or thousands of dollars worth of crack and will spend days smoking crack until all of it is used. Thus, it is unlikely that satiation explains the regularized reduction in cocaine/crack use on every Sunday.

4. *The Avoidance of Punishment Hypothesis.* As members of a methadone maintenance program, patients are given a urine test for drugs randomly during the week. However, patients do not go to the center on Sunday. Patients may develop the strategy of using cocaine on Saturday on the basis of the following expectations: (a) that the traces of cocaine may be cleared out of their system by Monday or (b) since there is only a one chance in six that they will be tested on Monday, its worth the risk. There is problem with this explanation. If patients were really concerned with detection, then patients would use cocaine on the day of urine testing, after having taken the test. At this point they know that there will be no other test for the rest of the week. Thus, being tested on Monday means that the subject has the rest of the week to use. However, if this were the case, then usage should not peak on Saturday; rather, because of the random pattern of testing over the week, cocaine use should be more or less uniform over the course of the week. Some patients may avoid using cocaine on Sunday because of fears of being detected on Monday but this would not explain why they would wait until Saturday to use when they could use immediately after having their urine test.

6. *The Cocaine Availability Hypothesis.* Cocaine is likely to be least available on Sundays and most available on Saturdays. Cocaine dealers congregate around methadone programs.[27] Therefore, during the six days of the week while the methadone program is open, methadone clients are exposed to dealers offering cocaine. Saturdays may be a day of even greater opportunity for using since this was the only day that study patients

pick up a "take-home" methadone dose. There is a ready blackmarket of methadone and cocaine-using methadone patients are more likely to sell their methadone dose than methadone patients who do not use cocaine.[28] Thus, it is possible that some of the patients sold their methadone on Saturdays and used the money received to purchase cocaine.

7. *The Conditioning Mechanisms Hypothesis.* A complex chain of operantly and classically conditioned stimuli and responses may serve as the basis for cocaine use, and exposure to the stimuli that elicit this chain varies from day to day. It is clear that certain kinds of stimulus conditions lead to drug use. In the present case, such STU variables as receiving money, being offered cocaine, and seeing cocaine and/or paraphernalia are significant predictors. But how do these variables operate? If they are classically conditioned stimuli, then we would expect that their occurrence would give rise to a conditioned responses of euphoria or withdrawal. This does not seem to be the case since no one reported this; in fairness though, patients were not explicitly asked. It seems more reasonable to think of STU variables as discriminative stimuli that signal the opportunity for cocaine use. In addition, it is possible that these STU variables are classically conditioned to internal states of distress which are interpreted as craving. They in turn increase the motivational state of the person to carry through the chain of events and responses leading to actual cocaine use, that is, the chain from exposure to cocaine or cocaine related stimuli to acquisition of cocaine to administration of cocaine to euphoric state. Regardless of the actual conditioning mechanisms, what is important is that the stimulus events triggering the chain of behavior vary from day to day and, as shown previously (see Table 3 and Figure 2), this appears to be the case in the current situation, that is, levels of STU variables vary from day to day with the lowest level of occurrence being Sunday. We propose that this account serves as a good tentative explanation of why cocaine use varies among the days of the week.

Note that this explanation is consistent with the social activity hypothesis (1 above) and the cocaine availability hypothesis (6 above). The cocaine availability explanation identifies certain environmental conditions, such as low availability on Sunday, but does not explain why a person would take advantage of these conditions to use cocaine on other days of the week. The question still remains why a person would use cocaine when it is available, and the conditioning mechanisms would serve as one explanation for why a person is motivated to use.

8. *The Cognitive Mechanisms Hypothesis.* Tiffany[13] has suggested viewing drug craving and use from the perspective of a cognitive model based on the operation of automatic and controlled processes.[15,16] The explana-

tion here would be comparable to that of conditioning, namely, that it is the variability in daily exposure to stimuli associated with cocaine use that causes the day of the week effect to occur, but differs in the type of mechanism that produces drug use behavior. Instead of operantly and classically conditioned stimulus and response conditions, certain stimuli trigger automatic cognitive processes that typically operate outside of conscious awareness (though manipulable by conscious action if one so desires) and produce behaviors that ultimately result in cocaine use. The specifics of how such a mechanism would, in fact, operate are beyond the scope of the current paper, but it does represent a reasonable alternative explanation to that based solely on conditioning mechanisms.

The results presented here raise many additional questions, such as what are the actual activities other than cocaine/crack use that patients engage in and how does this vary from day to day. Do cocaine users perceive craving, leading to a search for stimuli which signaled the availability of cocaine (i.e., craving driving drug-seeking and drug-using behavior), or did the mere occurrence of certain stimuli lead to craving, which served as the motivation for cocaine use (i.e., stimulus exposure leading to craving leading to drug seeking and drug use behavior)? It is even possible that the psychological construct of craving is unnecessary, that it is only an epiphenomenon, the by-product of a conditioned response to a STU or the activation of an automatic cognitive process. That the environments that these patients experienced on Sunday, along with the activities that they engaged in, were different from the rest of the week, would support the availability, conditioning, and cognitive accounts for why cocaine use is the lowest on Sunday. To develop a deeper understanding of the stimulus conditions to which these patients may have been exposed, and the activities that they may have engaged in, a study is being conducted which asks for detailed reporting on a daily basis for 7-10 days. It is hoped that this microlevel of analysis will provide additional specific information about the stimuli leading to cocaine use, whether craving has a direct or indirect effect, how often cocaine is used in a given day, and how these factors vary on a daily basis.

It is important to note that the present sample is drawn from a specific population, namely, patients in methadone maintenance with concurrent opiate/cocaine dependence. It is possible that studies of other populations, such as primary cocaine users may show different temporal patterns of usage. This is less of a concern than the identification of the contextual and psychological mechanisms that lead to cocaine use. If these mechanisms depend upon exposure to specific stimuli, and if these stimuli vary in their occurrence on a daily basis, then we should be able to predict on which days use will occur, simply from the knowledge of when the critical stimuli occur. It is quite possible that there are similar temporal patterns for other cocaine-using populations but it would not be surprising to find that some day other than Sunday has the lowest level of cocaine use.

REFERENCES

1. Johanson CE. Assessment of the dependence potential of cocaine in animals. NIDA Res Monogr 1984; 50: 54-71.

2. Childress AR, Hole AV, Ehrman RN, Robbins SJ, McLellan AT, O'Brien CP. Cue reactivity and cue reactivity interventions in drug dependence. NIDA Res Monogr 1993;137: 73-95.

3. Childress AR, McLellan AT, O'Brien CP. Conditioned responses in a methadone population: A comparison of laboratory, clinic, and natural settings. J Subst Abuse Treat 1986; 3:173-179.

4. O'Brien CP, Childress AR, McLellan AT, Ehrman R, Ternes JW. Types of conditioning found in drug-dependent humans. NIDA Res Monogr 1986; 84:44-61.

5. Rohenow DJ, Niaura RS, Childress AR, Abrams DB, et al. Cue reactivity in addictive behaviors: theoretical and treatment implications. Int J Addict 1990-1991;25:957-993.

6. Ehrman RN, Robbins SJ, Childress AR, O'Brien CP. Conditioned responses to cocaine-related stimuli in cocaine abuse. Psychopharmacology 1992; 107:523-529.

7. Robbins SJ, Ehrman RN, Childress AR, O'Brien CP. Using cue reactivity to screen medications for cocaine abuse: A test of amantadine hydrochloride. Addict Behav 1992; 17:491-499.

8. Childress AR, Ehrman R, McLellan AT, MacRae J, Natale M., O'Brien CP. Can induced moods trigger drug-related responses in opiate abuse patients? J Subst Abuse Treat 1994;11:17-23.

9. Childress AR, McLellan AT, Natale M, O'Brien CP. Mood states can elicit conditioned withdrawal and craving in opiate abuse patients. NIDA Res Monogr 1987;76:137-144.

10. Childress AR, McLellan AT, Ehrman RN, O'Brien CP. Extinction of conditioned responses in abstinent cocaine or opioid users. NIDA Res Monogr 1987; 76:189-195.

11. Childress AR, Ehrman R, McLellan AT, O'Brien CP. Update on behavioral treatments for substance abuse. NIDA Res Monogr 1988;90:183-192.

12. O'Brien CP, Childress AR, McLellan T, Ehrman R. Integrating systematic cue exposure with standard treatment in recovering drug dependent patients. Addict Behav 1990;15:355-365.

13. Tiffany ST. A cognitive model of drug urges and drug-use behavior: Role of automatic and nonautomatic processes. Psychol Rev 1990; 97:147-168.

14. Anderson JR. The adaptive character of thought. Hillsdale, NJ: Erlbaum, 1990.

15. Schneider W, Shiffrin RM. Controlled and automatic human information processing: I. Detection, search, and attention. Psychol Rev 1977;84:1-66.

16. Shiffrin RM, Schneider W. Controlled and automatic processing: II. Perceptual learning, automatic attending, and a general theory. Psychol Rev 1977;84:127-190.

17. Beck AT, Wright FD, Newman CF, Liese BS. Cognitive therapy of substance abuse. New York: Guilford, 1993.

18. Marlatt GA, Gordon JR. Relapse prevention: Maintenance strategies in the treatment of addictive behaviors. New York: Guilford, 1985.

19. Rawson RA, Obert JL, McCann MJ, Smith DP, Ling W. Neurobehavioral treatment for cocaine dependency. J Psychoactive Drugs 1990;22:159-171.

20. Magura S, Rosenblum A, Lovejoy M, Handelsman L, Foote J, Stimmel B. Neurobehavioral treatment for cocaine-using methadone patients: A preliminary report. J Addict Dis 1994; 13:143-160.

21. Handelsman L, Rosenblum A, Palij M, Magura S, Foote J, Lovejoy M, Stimmel B. Bromocriptine for cocaine dependence: A controlled clinical trial. Am J Addict; in press.

22. Rosenblum A, Magura S, Foote J, Palij M, Handelsman L, Lovejoy M, Stimmel B. Treatment intensity and reduction in drug use for cocaine-dependent methadone patients: a dose-response relationship. J Psychoactive Drugs 1995; 27:151-159.

23. Winer BJ. Statistical principles in experimental design (2nd ed.) New York: McGraw-Hill, 1971.

24. Aldrich JH, Nelson FD. Linear probability, logit, and probit models. Beverly Hills: Sage, 1984.

25. Palij M, Rosenblum A, Magura S, Handelsman L, Foote J, Lovejoy M. Daily patterns of cocaine abuse: Never on a Sunday? Poster presented at the Sixth Annual Meeting of the American Psychological Society, Washington, D. C., 1994.

26. Hosmer DW, Lemeshow S. Applied logistic regression. New York: Wiley, 1989.

27. Kolar AF, Brown BS, Weddington WW, Ball JC. A treatment crisis: cocaine use by clients in methadone maintenance. J Subst Abuse Treat 1990;7:101-107.

28. Spunt B, Hunt DE, Lipton DS, Goldsmith D. Methadone diversion: A new look. J Drug Issues, 1986, 16, 569-583.

Neurometric QEEG Studies
of Crack Cocaine Dependence
and Treatment Outcome

Leslie S. Prichep, PhD
Kenneth Alper, MD
Sharon C. Kowalik, MD, PhD
Mitchell Rosenthal, MD

SUMMARY. This paper presents an overview of the quantitative electrophysiological (QEEG) research on cocaine dependence conducted at Brain Research Laboratories of New York University Medical Center. These studies have demonstrated that subjects with DSM-III-R cocaine dependence (without dependence on any other substance) evaluated in the withdrawal state, have replicable abnormalities in brain function when evaluated at baseline (approximately

---

Leslie S. Prichep, Kenneth Alper, and Sharon C. Kowalik are affiliated with Brain Research Laboratories, Department of Psychiatry, New York University Medical Center, New York, NY. Leslie S. Prichep is also affiliated with the Nathan Kline Institute for Psychiatric Research, Orangeburg, NY.

Mitchell Rosenthal is affiliated with Phoenix House Foundation, New York, NY.

Address correspondence to: Leslie S. Prichep, PhD, Brain Research Laboratories, Department of Psychiatry, NYU Medical Center, 550 First Avenue, New York, NY 10016.

The authors gratefully acknowledge the contributions of Henry Merkin, MeeLee Tom and Larisa Vaysblat to this research.

This research was supported by the National Institute on Drug Abuse, Grant #RO1DA07707.

[Haworth co-indexing entry note]: "Neurometric QEEG Studies of Crack Cocaine Dependence and Treatment Outcome." Prichep, Leslie S. et al. Co-published simultaneously in *Journal of Addictive Diseases* (The Haworth Medical Press, an imprint of The Haworth Press, Inc.) Vol. 15, No. 4, 1996, pp. 39-53; and: *The Neurobiology of Cocaine Addiction: From Bench to Bedside* (ed: Herman Joseph, and Barry Stimmel) The Haworth Medical Press, an imprint of The Haworth Press, Inc., 1996, pp. 39-53. Single or multiple copies of this article are available for a fee from The Haworth Document Delivery Service [1-800-342-9678, 9:00 a.m. - 5:00 p.m. (EST). E-mail address: getinfo@haworth.com].

5 to 10 days after last crack cocaine use),[1,2] which are still seen at one and six month follow-up evaluations.[3] These abnormalities were characterized by significant excess of relative alpha power and deficit of absolute and relative delta and theta power. Abnormalities were greater in anterior than posterior regions, and disturbances in interhemispheric relationships were also observed. In addition, QEEG subtypes were identified within the population of cocaine dependent subjects at baseline, and these subtypes were found to be significantly related to subsequent length of stay in treatment. The relationship between these QEEG findings and the neuropharmacology of cocaine dependence is discussed. *[Article copies available for a fee from The Haworth Document Delivery Service: 1-800-342-9678. E-mail address: getinfo@haworth.com]*

INTRODUCTION

Electrophysiological investigations of the use of cocaine in adults suggest that the EEG is sensitive to the acute and chronic effects of cocaine.[1,2,4,5,6,7,8,9,10,11] Such changes may be related to the reported changes in neurotransmission following chronic exposure to cocaine.[12,13,14] The majority of existing QEEG studies in the literature report changes under acute administration of cocaine. In a study replicating Hans Berger's seminal work on the EEG in cocaine intoxication,[15] Herning et al. (1987, 1994) reported increased beta activity which was interpreted as an effect mediated by activation of the central noradrenergic arousal system. In a pilot study Lukas (1989), on the other hand, reported enhanced alpha correlating with self reported euphoria in subjects who administered cocaine intranasally. In these subjects, relatively low doses produced alpha but beta was observed with higher doses. The use of the intravenous route by Herning et al. (1987) and the observed dose response relationship noted by Lukas (1989) are possible explanations for these apparently divergent findings, and exemplify some of the methodological challenges inherent in studies involving acute cocaine administration.

The study of the quantitative EEG (QEEG) of adults in the drug free withdrawal state offers the opportunity to investigate changes in brain function following chronic exposure to cocaine. This review summarizes the studies done in our laboratory focusing on the QEEG changes in chronic crack cocaine dependent subjects, using a standardized, age regressed, method of quantification known as neurometrics.[18,19,20] In a pilot study of 7 chronic crack cocaine dependent subjects abstinent for 1 to 63 days, we reported significant excess absolute and relative alpha power and widespread deficits of absolute and relative power in the delta frequency band.[1] The subjects in this pilot study evidenced significant comorbid depression, and it was noted that increased alpha has been found in multiple independent studies of depressed patients.[21] Other QEEG findings observed in depression, however, such as decreased anterior coherence were not encountered, suggesting a distinction between uncomplicated cocaine abstinence from cocaine abstinence complicated by a major affective syndrome.[22]

The findings to be reviewed herein replicate and extend this initial pilot work. The methodology used in the studies to be described is given below.

SUBJECTS AND METHODS

These studies obtained approval from the New York University Medical Center's Institutional Board of Research Associates. Written informed consent was obtained from all subjects.

Subjects

Subjects were recruited from consecutive admissions to Phoenix House Foundation's Induction Facility in New York City. Phoenix House is a large drug-free therapeutic community, with multiple sites in the Northeastern US and California.

Psychiatric and neuropsychological evaluations were done on subjects who met the *Inclusion/Exclusion* criteria described below:

1. Fulfilling DSM-III-R criteria for cocaine dependence for at least one year and self report of strongly preferring crack cocaine to any other substance;
2. No history of having met DSM-III-R criteria for dependence on any other substance;
3. Alcohol intake limited to current levels which would not meet DSM-III-R dependence criteria;
4. Negative urine screening for other drugs;
5. No history of head trauma, neurologic or other significant medical condition;
6. No history of IV drug use;
7. No evidence of HIV infection;
8. No history of psychotropic medication treatment within 60 days of intake; and
9. IQs within the normal/low normal range (estimated IQs ≥ 80).

The results presented herein were based on the first 67 subjects who met intake criteria. This population consisted of 25 females and 42 males, with a mean age of 31.4 years (17.7-48.5 years). The distribution of these subjects by race was 77.6% Black, 14.9% Hispanic, and 7.5% Caucasian, which is consistent with the racial distribution of the Phoenix House population. Mean years of education was 11.5 (8-16); age of first crack use was 24.3 yrs. ± 6.4; number of years since first use of crack was 6.9 ± 3.4; weekly crack use over the past year was 5.1 g/wk ± 6.6; intensity of craving was 3.4 ± 3.3 using the Minnesota Cocaine Craving Scale.[23]

The self report of time since last crack use prior to entering Phoenix House was elicited in the absence of the subjects knowledge of the implication of his or her answer to study participation. Average time between reported date of last use of crack and date of entry to Phoenix House was 3.2 days (±2.4). Abstinence while in Phoenix House was verified by random urine testing.

EEG Data Acquisition

The patients were seated comfortably in a light attenuated room, while twenty minutes of eyes closed resting EEG data were collected from the 19 monopolar electrode sites of the International 10/20 system, referenced to linked earlobes. A differential eye channel was used for the detection of eye movement. All electrode impedances were below 5000Ω. The EEG amplifiers had a bandpass from 0.5 to 70 Hz (3 dB points), with a 60 Hz notch filter.

QEEG Data Analysis

Two minutes of artifact-free data were extracted from the EEG record for quantitative analysis. A computerized artifact-detection algorithm combined with visual inspection was used to obtain 48 epochs (2.5 sec each, for a total of 2 min) of artifact-free data from 20 min of continuous EEG. Power spectral analysis was performed using Fast Fourier Transform (FFT). For each of the 19 monopolar derivations, absolute and relative (%) power, mean frequency, inter- and intra-hemispheric coherence and symmetry were computed for the delta (1.5-3.5 Hz), theta (3.5-7.5 Hz), alpha (7.5 to 12.5 Hz), and beta (12.5-25 Hz) frequency bands. Using neurometrics quantitative features are log transformed to obtain Gaussianity, age-regressed, and Z-transformed relative to population norms. The importance of each of these steps in enhancing the sensitivity and specificity of electrophysiological data has been discussed in detail elsewhere,[24] as are test-retest reliability,[25,26,27] and independent replications of the Neurometric QEEG norms.[28,29,30,31,32,33,34] Color coded topographic maps of Z transformed data in standard deviation units can be displayed. Hotelling T^2's were computed to statistically assess the multivariate similarity between successive evaluations.

Length of Stay in Treatment

A variable for *length of stay in treatment* (LOST) was computed by subtracting the date the patient left the program from the date of entry to the program. The median length of stay (LOST) for subjects who had *already terminated* treatment was found to be 20 weeks. In this study, differential QEEG characteristics were sought between a "short stay" group which remained in treatment <20 weeks and a "long stay" group which had remained in treatment for ≥ 20 weeks. In order to take advantage of the largest population for study, it was determined that individuals who were still in the program, but had already completed ≥ 20 weeks of treatment could be added to the study population. That is, since the median length of stay was 20 weeks based on actual attrition and only baseline data was used in this study, if an individual completed 20 weeks then they were included for study.

Cluster Analysis

To identify the existence of homogeneous electrophysiological subtypes within the study population, cluster analysis was used (BMDP K-Means). A subset of 14 neurometric variables were selected for the cluster analysis. Variable selection was aided by use of *t*-tests and ANOVAs.[35]

RESULTS

Replication and Extension of Pilot Findings

The baseline QEEG findings in this population (N = 67), containing none of the subjects from the initial pilot study, replicated the neurophysiological profile reported in our published pilot study.[1,2] The group average baseline findings are summarized in Table 1 for each measure set in each brain region. Entries in this table are coded for the significance level of the finding taking the group size into account. As can be seen in this table, the QEEG profile in these subjects was characterized by significant deficits of absolute and relative power in the delta and theta frequency bands, and significant relative power excess in alpha. Mean frequency in the delta band was significantly increased globally, as was mean frequency in the theta band in frontal regions. Significant hypercoherence was seen between occipital regions in all bands, and between frontopolar regions in the theta, alpha, and beta bands. In addition, significant interhemispheric power asymmetries were seen in all bands, with more power on the right in frontal regions (FP1 vs FP2, and F7 vs F8), and more power on the left in occipital regions (O1 vs O2). In order to estimate how representative these results were for the group, standard deviations were computed for each measure set. All standard deviations were found to be between .5 and 1.6, suggesting that the group data was in fact representative of the group with little variance around the mean. Similar findings have been recently reported by Roemer et al. (1995) in subjects recovering from polysubstance abuse with preferential use of cocaine.

Length of exposure to crack cocaine was found to have significant positive correlations with mean frequency in theta, negative correlations with mean frequency in alpha, negative correlations with coherence between posterior regions (all bands), and positive correlations with coherence between anterior regions (theta and beta).

Persistence of QEEG Profile at Follow-Up (1-6 Months of Abstinence)

Comparisons between the neurometric profile of 39 patients at baseline and their neurometric profiles after one month of abstinence show remarkable stability. Figure 1 shows topographic Z maps for absolute (top row each panel) and relative power (bottom row each panel) at baseline (top panel) and after 1 month of abstinence (middle panel). Seventeen subjects from this group have now been in the program long enough to have been evaluated after 6 months of abstinence, and are shown in the bottom panel of this figure. Persistence of the baseline pattern can clearly be seen at these two follow-up intervals. Considering all variables, using the Hotelling T^2, statistically significant persistence of the profiles (i.e., no significant changes) was demonstrated at 1 and 6 month interval.[3,36] The persistence of this profile could suggest either that alterations in brain function following cocaine exposure are reflected in a neurometric profile which remains during abstinence for at least 6 months, or that the electrophysiological abnormalities reflect a "trait" related to vulnerability to crack cocaine addiction.

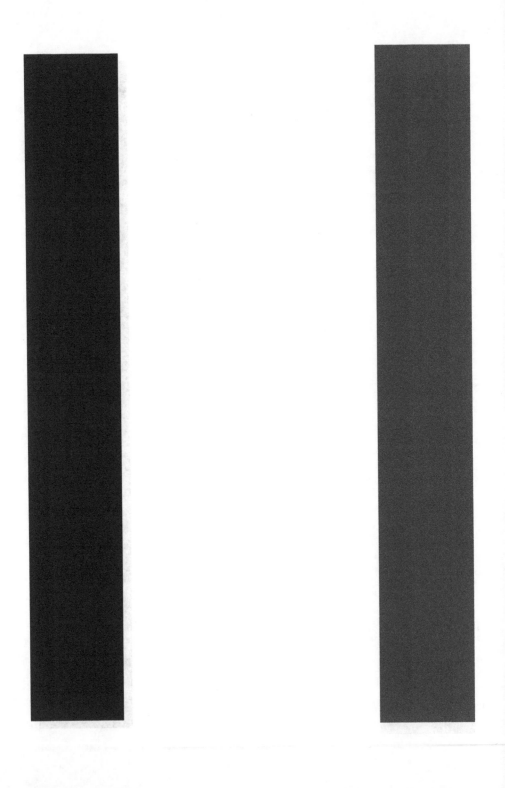

Correlates of Length of Stay in Treatment

For these analyses, the baseline evaluations of the population of 54 subjects was divided into two groups based on information about subsequent length of stay in treatment [LOST, <20 weeks or ≥20 weeks as described above (see METHODS)]. The first group contained 28 subjects (12 females, 16 males) who dropped out of treatment during the first 20 weeks (mean 7.5 weeks ± 5.8), and a second group of 26 patients (7 females, 19 males) who, at the time of this writing, had remained in treatment ≥20 weeks (mean 43.6 ± 20.5). No significant gender differences were seen in these distributions.

Using ANOVAs we explored the relationship between LOST and baseline QEEG features. Several highly significant findings (p ≤ 0.01) were obtained, suggesting a strong relationship between baseline neurometric QEEG features and subsequent LOST. These features include frontal bipolar frequency, symmetry and coherence features; monopolar beta relative power; monopolar mean frequency shifts in the total spectrum; and monopolar intrahemispheric asymmetry.

QEEG Prediction of Length of Stay in Treatment

Clear differences were seen in the baseline QEEG features of those who remain in treatment ≥20 weeks and <20 weeks. In general, those who leave treatment earlier show significantly more alpha, less delta and theta, and more alpha hypercoherence. Based on these suggestive findings, we used cluster analysis of the baseline QEEG features to search for subtypes defined without prior knowledge of outcome. This study is described in detail elsewhere,[37,38] but is summarized briefly below.

The variance attributed to gender could not be reliably estimated from the small number of female subjects available at the time of these analyses. Thus, 35 male subjects, with an average age of 32.0 years (age range of 17.7-48.5 years) were included in this study. Neurometric evaluations were done 5-10 days after last reported cocaine use.

A small subset of QEEG baseline variables were submitted to cluster analysis to determine whether subtypes could be identified. Two clusters were described, one characterized by significant deficits of delta and theta with excess of alpha, and the second by deficits of delta, more normal theta and alpha, and excess of beta. While no significant relationships were found between subtype membership and any demographic or clinical characteristics, a significant relationship (p ≤ 0.003) between QEEG subtype and length of stay in treatment (continued abstinence) was found. 81.3% of Cluster 1 members remained in treatment less than

20 weeks, and 84.2% of Cluster 2 members remained in treatment more than 20 weeks. It is of interest to note that when the females are clustered using the algorithm derived from the males, those who remain in treatment are well predicted, but not those who leave treatment early. This suggests that there are greater differences in the early termination group and implies the need for further exploration in a larger group of female subjects.

Encouraged by the little overlap between the LOST distributions of the two clusters, we attempted a preliminary regression analysis (SAS-PROC REG) to study more precisely the degree to which a small subset of QEEG baseline features can be used to mathematically predict length of stay in treatment. Although considered preliminary in nature, thirteen QEEG baseline variables were used to derive a regression equation with an $r^2 =$ .81 (p ≤ 0.0001) for the population. The variables which predicted the greatest percentage of variance were predominantly bipolar, frequently multivariates (composite features with intercorrelation removed), and shifts in mean frequencies in slow waves. However, it was observed that the mean errors of prediction were higher for the females than for the males, suggesting that the disproportionate number of males made this a sub-optimal predictor. Further, this suggests the possibility of significant gender interactions between LOST and QEEG.

DISCUSSION

The results of the studies reviewed herein are described in the context of current hypotheses of sensitization in the pathophysiology of cocaine dependence. A current hypothesis regarding the neurobiology of cocaine dependence attributes an important role to the sensitization of dopaminergic (DA) cells in the ventral tegmental area (VTA).[14,39,40] Repeated administration of cocaine sensitizes the response of VTA DA neurons to DA agonists and a number of other activating conditions such as stress, administration of corticosterone, "priming" doses of rewarding substances, or the presentation of conditioned cues.[14,39,41,42] The time course of sensitization, which can be months to years (unlike reported changes in DA transmission associated with tolerance which appears to resolve within a few days or weeks of abstinence[14,43]), is consistent with our report of persistent abnormalities in the QEEG across the time span studied.

The fact that stimulation or DA administration to the VTA desynchronizes slow EEG activity[44] is consistent with the observed slow wave *deficit* in cocaine dependence. Although deficits of slow waves historically have not been clinically interpreted, delta deficits have been reported in multiple studies of cocaine dependent patients, suggesting that it be considered independently of the increase in alpha. In fact, absolute power findings in these studies support the relative independence of power in the alpha and delta bandwidths. There is also a substantial literature relating delta power increases to higher order mental functions in normal humans. Increased delta activity has been observed in normal subjects performing calculations,[45] reaction time tasks,[46] abstract thought,[47] an omitted stimulus paradigm,[48] and to correlate positively with P300 amplitude.[49] Fernandez et al. (1995) postulate that the functional role of such increased delta may be "inner-concentration," suppressing extraneous inputs in order to allocate maximal attention. A deficit of this "physiologic delta" may reflect a failure to normally gate maladaptive behavior or extraneous cues, and is therefore logically consistent with expectation of a greater determination of behavior by limbic relative to frontal cortical input in the sensitization models of cocaine dependence.[14,42] Also of note is that the clinical populations in our database with delta deficits include attention deficit hyperactivity disorder (ADHD),[50] subtypes of obsessive compulsive disorder (OCD)[51] and subtypes of schizophrenia,[52] all of which are noted to have impairments with respect to the ability to gate preattentive or extraneous stimuli.

The finding of increased alpha is of interest in view of the tendency of antidepressants to diminish alpha.[21,53] Antidepressants have been used to treat cocaine dependence.[54] The expected effect of an antidepressant in cocaine withdrawal would be to make the power spectrum relatively more normal, which is similar in concept to the "corrective function" proposed for antidepressants in reversing the alpha excess typically seen in depression.[21]

The spectral power profile we and others have observed in cocaine dependence differs substantially from those reported in alcohol,[21] cannabis[55,56] and HIV,[57] suggesting a degree of specificity of the findings. In addition, the apparent relationship of baseline QEEG to subsequent retention in treatment if replicated, provides evidence of specificity in the form of a correlation of the QEEG with a cardinal feature of cocaine dependence, the tendency to relapse after years to months of abstinence. In view of the reported lack of predictive ability of sociodemographic or clinical behavioral measures, the data presented here support the possibility that QEEG can play a potentially useful role in drug development and treatment planning, as well as in the understanding of the pathophysiology of cocaine dependence.

REFERENCES

1. KR Alper, RJ Chabot, AH Kim, LS Prichep, and ER John. Quantitative EEG correlates of crack cocaine dependence. Psychiat. Res., 35:95-106, 1990.

2. LS Prichep, KR Alper, SC Kowalik, ER John, HA Merkin, M Tom, and MS Rosenthal. Quantitative electroencephalographic characteristics of crack cocaine dependence. Biol. Psychiat., (In Press), 1996.

3. KR Alper, LS Prichep, MS Rosenthal, ER John, M Tom, and HA Merkin. Persistence of QEEG abnormality in crack cocaine withdrawal. In Abstracts from the College on Problems of Drug Dependence, Scottsdale, AZ, 1995.

4. RI Herning, RT Jones, WD Hooker, J Mendelson, and L Blackwell. Cocaine increases EEG beta: A replication and extension of Hans Berger's historic experiments. EEG Clin. Neurophysiol., 60:470-477, 1985.

5. SE Lukas, JH Mendelson, BT Woods, NK Mello, and SK Teoh. Topographic distribution of EEG alpha activity during ethanol-induced intoxication in women. J. Studies on Alcohol, 50(2):176-184, 1989.

6. A Dhuna, A Pascual-Leone, F Langendorf, and DC Anderson. Epileptogenic properties of cocaine in humans. Neurotoxicology, 12:621-626, 1991.

7. A Pascual-Leone, A Dhuna, and DS Anderson. Longterm neurological complications of chronic habitual cocaine abuse. Neurotoxicology, 12:393-400, 1991.

8. A Cornwell, RA Roemer, DB Dewart, and P Jackson. Paroxysmal EEG activity in cocaine abstinence. NIDA Research Monograph, 141(163), 1993.

9. RA Roemer, A Cornwell, DB Dewart, and P Jackson. Quantitative QEEG analyses in cocaine abstinent subjects. NIDA Research Monograph, 141(33), 1993.

10. NE Noldy, CV Santos, N Politzer, RDG Blair, and PL Carlen. Quantitative EEG changes in cocaine withdrawal: Evidence for long-term CNS effects. Neuropsychobiology, 30, 1994.

11. RA Roemer, A Cornwall, D Dewart, P Jackson, and DV Ercegovac. Quantitative electroencephalographic analysis in cocaine-preferring polysubstance abusers during abstinence. Psychiat. Res., 58:247-257, 1995.

12. ND Volkow, R Hitzemann, G Wang, JS Fowler, AP Wolf, SL Dewey, and L Handleman. Long-term frontal brain metabolic changes in cocaine abusers. Synapse, 11:184-190, 1992.

13. EJ Nestler. Molecular neurobiology of drug addiction. Neuropsychopharmacology, 11(2):77-87, 1994.

14. AA Grace. The tonic/phasic model of dopamine system regulation: its relevance for understanding how stimulant abuse can alter basal ganglia function. Drug Alc. Depend., 37:111-129, 1995.

15. HA Berger. Electroencephalogram of man. Arch. Psychiat. Nervenkr., 106:577-584, 1937.

16. RI Herning, WD Hooker, and RT Jones. Cocaine effects on electroencephalographic cognitive event-related potentials and performance. EEG Clin. Neurophysiol, 66:34-42, 1987.

17. RI Herning, BJ Glover, B Koeppl, RL Phillips, and ED London. Cocaine-induced increases in EEG alpha and beta activity: Evidence for reduced cortical processing. Neuropsychopharmacol., 11(1):1-9, 1994.

18. ER John, H Ahn, LS Prichep, M Trepetin, D Brown, and H Kaye. Developmental equations for the electroencephalogram. Science, 210:1255-1258, 1980.

19. LS Prichep and ER John. Neurometrics: Clinical applications. In FH Lopes da Silva, W Storm van Leeuwen, and A Remond, editors, Clinical Applications of Computer Analysis of EEG and Other Neurophysiological Variables, volume 2 of Handbook of Electroencephalography and Clinical Neurophysiology, pages 153-170. Elsevier, Amsterdam, 1986.

20. ER John, LS Prichep, J Fridman, and P Easton. Neurometrics: Computer assisted differential diagnosis of brain dysfunctions. Science, 293:162-169, 1988.

21. K Alper. Quantitative EEG and Evoked Potentials in Adult Psychiatry. In J Panksepp, editor, Advances in Biological Psychiatry, Vol. 1, pages 65-112. JAI Press, Greenwich, Connecticut, 1995.

22. KR Alper, R Chabot, LS Prichep, and ER John. Crack cocaine dependence: Discrimination from major depression using QEEG variables. In K. Maurer, editor, Imaging of the Brain in Psychiatry and Related Fields, pages 289-293. Springer-Verlag, Berlin, 1993.

23. JA Halikas, KL Kuhn, R Crosby, G Carlson, and F Crea. The measurements of craving in cocaine patients using the Minnesota Cocaine Craving Scale. Comp. Psychiat., 32:22-27, 1991.

24. ER John, LS Prichep, J Friedman, and T Essig-Peppard. Neurometric classification of patients with different psychiatric disorders. In D Samson-Dollfus, editor, Statistics and Topography in Quantitative EEG, pages 88-95. Elsevier, Paris, 1988.

25. H Kaye, ER John, H Ahn, and LS Prichep. Neurometric evaluation of learning disabled children. Intl. J. Neuroscience, 13:15-25, 1981.

26. ER John, LS Prichep, H Ahn, P Easton, J Fridman, and H Kaye. Neurometric evaluation of cognitive dysfunctions and neurological disorders in children. Progress in Neurobiol., 21:239-290, 1983.

27. G Fein, D Galin, CD Yingling, J Johnstone, and MA Nelson. EEG spectra in 9-13-year-old boys are stable over 1-3 years. EEG Clin. Neurophysiol, 58:517-518, 1984.

28. M Matousek and I Petersén. Norms for the EEG. In P Kellaway and I Petersén, editors, Automation of Clinical Electroencephalography, pages 75-102. Raven, New York, 1973.

29. T Gasser, P Bacher, and J Mochs. Transformation towards the normal distribution of broadband spectral parameters of the EEG. EEG Clin. Neurophysiol., 53:119-124, 1982.

30. EJ Jonkman, DCJ Poortvliet, MM Veering, AW deWeerd, and ER John. The use of neurometrics in the study of patients with cerebral ischemia. EEG Clin. Neurophysiol, 61:333-341, 1985.

31. CD Yingling, D Galin, G Fein, D Peltzman, and L Davenport. Neurometrics does not detect 'pure' dyslexics. EEG Clin. Neurophysiol., 63:426-430, 1986.

32. A Alvarez, R Pascual, and P Valdes. U. S. EEG developmental equations confirmed for Cuban schoolchildren. EEG Clin. Neurophysiol, 67:330-332, 1987.

33. T Harmony, A Alvarez, R Pascual, A Ramos, E Marosi, AE Diaz De Leon, P Valdes, and J Becker. EEG maturation of children with different economic and psychosocial characteristics. Intl. J. Neurosci., 31:103-113, 1987.

34. ER John, LS Prichep, H Ahn, H Kaye, D Brown, P Easton, BZ Karmel, A Toro, and R Thatcher. Neurometric Evaluation of Brain Function in Normal and Learning Disabled Children. Univ. of Michigan Press, Ann Arbor, 1989.

35. JM Weiner and OJ Dunn. Elimination of variates in linear discrimination problems. Biometrics, 22:268-275, 1966.

36. KR Alper, LS Prichep, SC Kowalik, L Vaysblat, and MS Rosenthal. Persistent quantitative EEG abnormalities in crack cocaine abstinence. Submitted to Arch. Gen. Psychiat., 1995.

37. LS Prichep, KR Alper, S Kowalik, L Vaysblat, HA Merkin, M Tom, ER John, and MS Rosenthal. Prediction of treatment outcome in crack cocaine dependence: Quantitative EEG and comorbidity. Drug Alc. Depend., (Accepted with revision), 1996.

38. LS Prichep, KR Alper, SC Kowalik, ER John, HA. Merkin, M. Tom, and MS Rosenthal. QEEG subtypes in crack cocaine dependence and treatment outcome. In In Abstracts, College on Problems of Drug Dependence 57th Annual Meeting, Scottsdale, AZ, page 114, 1995.

39. PW Kalivas, BA Sorg, and MS Hooks. The pharmacology and neural circuitry of sensitization to psychostimulants. Behav. Pharmacol., 4:315-334, 1993.

40. RH Roth and JD Elsworth. Biochemical pharmacology of midbrain dopamine neurons. In FE Bloom and DJ Kupfer, editors, Psychopharmacology: The Fourth Generation of Progress, chapter 21, pages 227-243. Raven Press, New York, 1995.

41. EA Kiyatkin. Functional significance of mesolimbic dopamine. Neurosci. Biobehav. Rvs., 19(4):578-598, 1995.

42. TE Robinson and KC Berridge. The neural basis of drug craving: An incentive-sensitization theory of addiction. Brain Res. Rvs., 18:247-291, 1993.

43. C-E Johanson and CR Schuster. Cocaine. In FE Bloom and DJ Kupfer, editors, Psychopharmacology: The Fourth Generation of Progress, chapter 145, pages 1685-1697. Raven Press, New York, 1995.

44. A Rougeul-Buser. Electrocortical rhythms in the 40 hz Band in cat: In search of their behavioral correlates. In G Buzsaki, R Llinas, W Singer, A Berthoz, and Y Christen, editors, Temporal Coding in the Brain, pages 103-114. Springer-Verlag, Berlin, 1994.

45. T Fernandez, T Harmony, M Rodriguez, J Bernal, J Silva, A Reyes, and E Marosi. EEG activation patterns during the performance of tasks involving different components of mental calculation. EEG Clin. Neurophysiol., 94:175-182, 1995.

46. JG Van Dijk, JFV Caekebeke, A Jennekens Schinkel, and AH Zwinderman. Background EEG reactivity in auditory event-related potentials. EEG Clin. Neurophysiol, 83:44-51, 1992.

47. CM Michel, B Henggeler, D Brandeis, and D Lehmann. Localization of sources of brain alpha/theta/delta activity and the influence of the mode spontaneous mentation. Physiol. Meas., 14:21-26, 1993.

48. C Basar-Eroglu, E Basar, T Demiralp, and M Schurmann. P300-response: possible psychophysioilogical correlates in delta and theta frequency channels. A review. Intl. J. Psychphysiol., 13:161-179, 1992.

49. J Intriligator and J Polich. On the relationship between background EEG and the P300 event-related potential. Biol. Psychiat., 37:207-218, 1994.

50. RJ Chabot and G Serfontein. Quantitative EEG profiles of children with Attention Deficit Disorder. Biol. Psychiat., (In press), 1996.

51. LS Prichep, F Mas, E Hollander, M Liebowitz, ER John, M Almas, CM DeCaria, and RH Levine. Quantitative electroencephalographic (QEEG) subtyping of obsessive compulsive disorder. Psychiat. Res., 50(1):25-32, 1993.

52. ER John, LS Prichep, KR Alper, FG Mas, R Cancro, P Easton, and L Sverdlov. Quantitative electrophysiological characteristics and subtyping of schizophrenia. Biol. Psychiat., 36:801-826, 1994.

53. TM Itil. The discovery of antidepressant drugs by computer-analyzed human cerebral bio-electrical potentials (CEEG). Progress in Neurobiol., 20:185-249, 1983.

54. FH Gwain, D Allen, and B Humbelstone. Outpatient treatment of 'crack' cocaine smoking with flupenthixol decanoate. Arch. Gen. Psychiat., 46: 322-325, 1989.

55. FA Struve, JJ Straumanis, G Patrick, and L Price. Topographic mapping of quantitative EEG variables in chronic heavy marijuana users: Empirical findings with psychiatric patients. Clin. EEG, 20(1):6-23, 1989.

56. FA Struve, JJ Straumanis, and G Patrick. Persistent topographic quantitative EEG sequelae of chronic marijuana use: A replication study and initial discriminant function analysis. Clin EEG, 25(2):63-75, 1994.

57. R-R Riedel, KR Alper, P Bulau, D Niese, U Schieck, and W Gunther. QEEG in hemophiliacs infected with HIV. Clin. EEG, 26:84-91, 1995.

Cocaine Addiction: Hypothesis Derived from Imaging Studies with PET

Nora D. Volkow, MD
Yu-Shin Ding, PhD
Joanna S. Fowler, PhD
Gene-Jack Wang, MD

SUMMARY. Analysis of the behavior of cocaine in the human brain with Positron Emission Tomography reveals that it is not only its affinity for the dopamine transporter that gives it its unique properties but also its fast pharmacokinetics. Its very fast uptake and clearance

---

Nora D. Volkow, Yu-Shin Ding, Joanna S. Fowler, and Gene-Jack Wang are affiliated with the Medical and Chemistry Departments, Brookhaven National Laboratory, Upton, NY. Nora D. Volkow is also affiliated with the Department of Psychiatry, State University of New York Stony Brook, Stony Brook, NY.

Address correspondence to: Nora D. Volkow, MD, Medical Department, Brookhaven National Laboratory, Upton, NY 11973.

The authors thank Robert Carciello and Babe Barrett for Cyclotron operations; Alex Levy and Donald Warner for PET operations; Colleen Shea, Robert MacGregor and Payton King for radiotracer preparation and analysis; Naomi Pappas, Kathy Pascani and Gail Burr for subject evaluation; Noelwah Netusil for patient care; Christopher Wong for data management; and Carol Redvanly for scheduling and organization.

This research was supported in part by the U.S. Department of Energy under Contract DE-ACO2-76CH00016 and NIDA Grants No. 5RO1-DA06891 and No. 1RO1-DA09490-01.

[Haworth co-indexing entry note]: "Cocaine Addiction: Hypothesis Derived from Imaging Studies with PET." Volkow, Nora D. et al. Co-published simultaneously in *Journal of Addictive Diseases* (The Haworth Medical Press, an imprint of The Haworth Press, Inc.) Vol. 15, No. 4, 1996, pp. 55-71; and: *The Neurobiology of Cocaine Addiction: From Bench to Bedside* (ed: Herman Joseph, and Barry Stimmel) The Haworth Medical Press, an imprint of The Haworth Press, Inc., 1996, pp. 55-71. Single or multiple copies of this article are available for a fee from The Haworth Document Delivery Service [1-800-342-9678, 9:00 a.m. - 5:00 p.m. (EST). E-mail address: getinfo@haworth.com].

from the brain contrasts with that of methylphenidate, another drug that inhibits the DA transporter. Methylphenidate clears from the brain at a much slower rate and is less addictive than cocaine. We postulate that periodic and frequent stimulation of the dopaminergic system secondary to chronic use of cocaine favors activation of a circuit that involves the orbitofrontal cortex, cingulate gyrus, thalamus and striatum. This circuit is abnormal in cocaine abusers and we postulate that its activation by cocaine perpetuates the compulsive administration of the drug and is perceived by the cocaine abuser as a intense desire resulting in the loss of control over the drive to take more cocaine. *[Article copies available for a fee from The Haworth Document Delivery Service: 1-800-342-9678. E-mail address: getinfo@ haworth.com]*

INTRODUCTION

The problem of cocaine addiction has to be understood both with respect to the properties of cocaine that make it such a reinforcing drug as well as the characteristics of the individuals who becomes addicted to it. Though it is well recognized that cocaine is among the most reinforcing of the drugs of abuse,[1,2] only 10-15% of those who initially try cocaine intranasally become cocaine abusers.[3] This highlights the importance of individual biological as well as environmental factors in cocaine addiction. Though it is also true that under experimental conditions where cocaine is freely available most animals will self-administer it at the exclusion of other behaviors,[3] these conditions are rarely those encountered in our society were cocaine is not only a illegal drug but is also expensive. Thus the question that remains to be answered is what are the mechanisms that will make an individual overcome the normal positive and negative societal reinforcers in favor of cocaine sometimes even at the expense of his or her own conscious will.[4]

In this paper we postulate that the unique pharmacological properties of cocaine serve as the link that triggers a pathological activation of a cerebral circuit that enables maintenance of behaviors that are required in order to achieve a targeted biological goal. This circuit which includes the orbitofrontal cortex, thalamus and striatum is involved in behaviors that require a repetitive pattern to achieve fulfillment of their biological goal such as eating, drinking, grooming and mating.[5] These behaviors are terminated either by satiety and/or competing distracting stimuli with consequent deactivation of this circuit. We hypothesize that cocaine addicts have a lower threshold for activation of this circuit by cocaine and that disruption of dopaminergic neurotransmission is in part responsible for this abnormality. Dysfunction of this circuit could result from either chronic use of cocaine or as a resultant of a biological characteristic that places subjects at risk for drug addiction. In this paper we discuss the results obtained from positron emission tomography (PET) studies that have led us to this hypothesis. PET studies were done to investigate the properties of cocaine in the living human brain and to assess brain function and dopamine brain activity in cocaine abusers.

PET is an imaging technique which allows the measurement of the concentration of positron-emitter labeled compounds in the living brain noninvasively.[6] Because the short-lived positron emitters such as carbon-11 (half-life: 20.4 minutes) can be used to label organic compounds without affecting their pharmacological properties, PET can be used to assess neurochemistry and pharmacology of the human brain. For example, PET has been used to evaluate the effects of acute cocaine on brain glucose metabolism[7] and the effects of chronic cocaine on cerebral blood flow,[8] glucose metabolism during early[9] and late[10] cocaine withdrawal, DA metabolism,[11] and DA D_2 receptor availability[12,13] as well as to assess the pharmacokinetics and distribution of cocaine[14] and cocaethylene (a metabolite from cocaine and ethanol) in the human brain[15] with and without alcohol intoxication,[16] and to compare it with the pharmacokinetics of methylphenidate[17] and to assess the distribution of ^{11}C cocaine in the human body.[18]

MATERIALS AND METHODS

Pharmacological Studies of Cocaine

Two strategies were used. The first strategy was to characterize cocaine binding in the baboon brain and to investigate its pharmacokinetics in the human brain.[14] The second strategy was to compare its behavior with that of methylphenidate,[17] a drug which, like cocaine, inhibits the dopamine transporter, (Ki for inhibition of dopamine uptake corresponds to 640 nM for cocaine and 390 nM for methylphenidate)[19] but which is abused in humans much less frequently than cocaine.[20]

Studies characterizing the binding of cocaine and methylphenidate were done in anesthetized baboons using PET and ^{11}C-cocaine and ^{11}C-methylphenidate, respectively. Details about the procedures have been published.[14,21] Briefly, baboons were scanned twice; first at baseline and then after preadministration of drugs that inhibit one of the monoamine transporters. Studies were also done with preadministration of pharmacological doses of cocaine (2 mg/kg iv.) and of methylphenidate (0.5 mg/kg iv.) to assess the ability of each one of these drugs to inhibit the binding of the other.

Studies on the pharmacokinetics of ^{11}C-cocaine and ^{11}C-methylphenidate were done in 10 and 8 healthy controls, respectively. One subject was tested twice, once with ^{11}C-cocaine and the second time with ^{11}C-methylphenidate. Details and procedures have been published.[14,17]

Studies on Cocaine Addicts

Two studies were done; one evaluated subjects during early cocaine withdrawal (<1 week) and involved studies in 15 outpatient chronic cocaine abusers and 14 normal controls[9,12] and the other was a longitudinal study that assessed the effects of protracted withdrawal at ~1 month and then after 4 months of detoxification and involved studies in 22 inpatient cocaine abusers and 24 normal controls.[10,13]

These studies involved chronic cocaine addicts that fulfilled DSM-III-R criteria for cocaine addiction as well as healthy non-abusing subjects as controls. Cocaine addicts had to consume at least 4 grams of cocaine a weeks for at least the 6 months that preceded the investigation and were excluded if they were dependent on other drugs of abuse (except caffeine and nicotine).

Subjects were tested with [18]FDG to measure regional brain glucose metabolism and with ^{18}F-NMS to assess dopamine D_2 receptors. For the longitudinal studies the scans were repeated 3 months after completion of an inpatient rehabilitation program. Details on scanning procedures as well as subjects characterization have been published.[9,10]

RESULTS

Pharmacological Studies

Cocaine binding in the brain was heterogeneous with the highest concentration in the striatum. Pretreatment with pharmacological doses of cocaine inhibited binding in the striatum but not in the cerebellum. Binding in the striatum was also inhibited by drugs that inhibited the dopamine transporter but not by drugs that inhibited the norepinephrine or the serotonin transporter.[14]

Studies of its pharmacokinetics in the human brain revealed a very fast uptake in the brain which occurred approximately 4-6 minutes after injection. At peak the concentration in the brain corresponded to 8-10% of the injected dose. The distribution in the brain was as for the baboon with the highest concentration in the striatum followed by the thalamus, cingulate gyrus, temporal cortex, frontal and occipital cortexes and cerebellum. Cocaine cleared very rapidly from the brain with a half-peak clearance in basal ganglia of approximately 20 minutes.[14]

Characterization studies with ^{11}C-methylphenidate revealed a similar binding profile to that observed with ^{11}C-cocaine (Figure 1). Maximal uptake was observed in the striatum where binding was inhibited by drugs that inhibited the DA transporter but not by drugs that inhibited the norepinephrine or the serotonin transporter.[21]

To assess binding overlap at the dopamine transporter between cocaine and methylphenidate we assessed the effects of pharmacological doses of methylphenidate on ^{11}C-cocaine binding and the effects of pharmacological doses of cocaine on ^{11}C-methylphenidate binding in the baboon brain. Both of these drugs inhibited the binding of the other in the striatum but not in the cerebellum indicating binding to the same or to an overlapping site.[17]

Studies on the pharmacokinetics of ^{11}C-methylphenidate revealed a fast uptake into the brain, with peak occurring 8-10 minutes after injection. At peak the concentration in brain corresponded to 7-9% of injected dose. Following the peak, the concentration of methylphenidate in basal ganglia plateaued for approximately 20-30 minutes and then cleared slowly for a half-life of approximately 90 minutes.[17]

To compare the kinetics of these two drugs in human brain we averaged the time activity curves for ^{11}C-cocaine and for ^{11}C-methylphenidate in striatum and cerebellum in the subjects investigated, (Figure 2). The values for peak uptake of ^{11}C-cocaine and of ^{11}C-methylphenidate in whole brain (global), in striatum and in cerebellum are shown in Table 1 along with the times to reach peak uptake and half peak clearance. Both drugs showed a similar rate of uptake in the brain but a much slower rate of clearance for ^{11}C-methylphenidate than for ^{11}C-cocaine. Despite the significant rate of clearance between these two drugs the duration of the high after their intravenous injection was of similar duration.[17]

In the case of cocaine the "high" as reported by Cook et al.[22] followed a parallel temporal course to that of ^{11}C-cocaine in the striatum (Figure 3). The "high" after intravenous injection of methylphenidate (0.5 mg/kg iv.) paralleled the fast rate of uptake of the drug in the brain of ^{11}C-methylphenidate but it declined rapidly despite the continuous binding of ^{11}C-methylphenidate in the brain (Figure 3).[17]

Studies in Cocaine Addicts

Regional brain glucose metabolism in recently detoxified cocaine abusers (< 1 week) was significantly higher in the orbitofrontal cortex and in the striatum than in healthy non-abusing controls and it was also (though not significant) higher than in the 5 cocaine abusers tested 2-4 weeks after withdrawal (Figure 4).[9] The metabolic activity in these brain regions was found to be correlated with the days since last use of cocaine. The highest values were observed in subjects tested during the initial 72 hours. Metabolic activity in the orbitofrontal cortex and in the striatum was significantly correlated with the intensity of cocaine craving. Cocaine abusers who had the highest subjective ratings for craving were those with the highest metabolic values in orbitofrontal cortex and striatum.[9] Studies done with ^{18}F-NMS on these same cocaine abusers revealed decreases in dopamine D_2 receptor availability.

In contrast to the marked increases in metabolism observed during early cocaine withdrawal, the study done in patients tested between 1 and 4 months of detoxification showed significant reductions in metabolic activity. These patients showed significant decrements in metabolism of the prefrontal cortex, orbito frontal cortex, temporal cortex and cingulate gyrus.[10] There were no changes in metabolic activity of the striatum. Measures of dopamine D_2 receptor availability showed a significant reduction as had been observed for the study in the patients tested during early detoxification.[13] Measures for D_2 receptors were not found to correlate with intensity of cocaine craving.[13] However, they were found to show a significant negative correlation with the subjective experience of dysphoria as assessed with the Beck depression inventory (Figure 5).[13] The measures of dopamine D_2 receptors in the cocaine abusers were also significantly correlated with measures of metabolic activity in the orbito frontal cortex, cingulate gyrus and prefrontal cortex (Figure 6).[13]

The decrements in regional brain metabolism as well as the reductions in dopamine D_2 receptor availability persisted in the follow up studies performed 3 months after completing the inpatient detoxification program.

DISCUSSION

These studies reveal the unique pharmacokinetics of cocaine when compared with that of methylphenidate, a drug with a similar affinity for the dopamine transporter but which is infrequently abused.[20] These differences were not in their rate of uptake but in their rate of clearance. Cocaine

FIGURE 3. Time activity curves for ^{11}C-cocaine in striatum (n = 10) and for ^{11}C-methylphenidate (n = 4) superimposed with the temporal changes on the "high" experienced after intravenous cocaine. The "high" from intravenous cocaine followed a parallel temporal course to that of ^{11}C-cocaine in the striatum. The "high" after intravenous methylphenidate paralleled the fast rate of uptake of ^{11}C-methylphenidate in the brain but it declined rapidly despite the continuous binding of ^{11}C-methylphenidate in the striatum. From Volkow et al.[17]

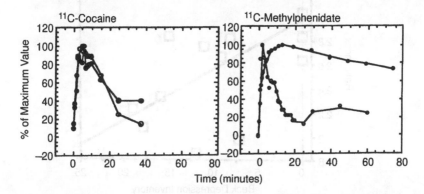

FIGURE 4. Individual regional brain metabolic values in the orbitofrontal cortex and in the striatum in 14 healthy controls (NML) and 14 cocaine abusers. Nine of the cocaine abusers were tested within one week of last use of cocaine (< 1W) and five between 2 and 4 weeks of last cocaine use (2-4W). Cocaine abusers tested during early cocaine withdrawal showed significantly higher metabolic values in the orbitofrontal cortex and striatum than normal controls.

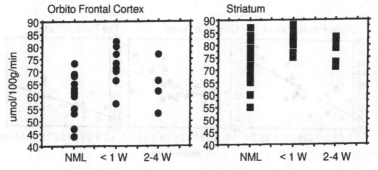

FIGURE 5. Correlation between the measures of dopamine D_2 receptors (Ratio Index) as assessed with PET and ^{18}F-NMS and the subjective experience of dysphoria as assessed with the Beck depression inventory in 17 of the cocaine abusers tested between 4 and 6 weeks after last cocaine use; r = 0.7 p < 0.002.

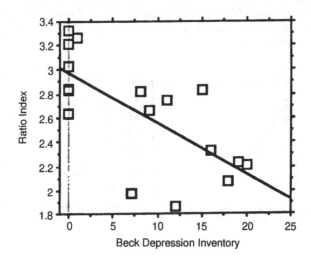

FIGURE 6. Correlation between the measures of dopamine D_2 receptors (Ratio Index) as assessed with PET and ^{18}F-NMS and measures of metabolic activity in the orbito frontal cortex, cingulate gyrus and prefrontal cortex in 22 cocaine abusers tested after protracted withdrawal (> 1 week, < 6 weeks).

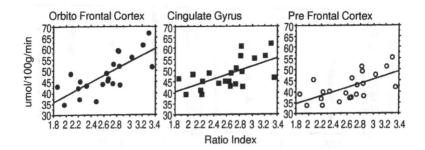

cleared from brain much faster than methylphenidate.[17] We believe that the fast pharmacokinetics of cocaine at the dopamine transporter account for its unique behavior when compared with that of other drugs that inhibit the dopamine transporter. Its high and fast rate of uptake accounts for its highly reinforcing properties and its fast clearance promotes its repeated and frequent self-administration. We believe that the pleasurable response experienced after cocaine and/or methylphenidate use, which is linked to the release of dopamine in the nucleus accumbens,[23] activates the orbito-frontal-thalamo-striatal circuit setting out the drive to continue to self-administer the drug, a state which is subjectively experienced as drug craving.[24] Other reinforcing drugs, such as methylphenidate[25,26,27] which clear slowly from brain,[16] may not be as effective in maintaining rapid and frequent administration and may therefore be less likely to induce binge-ing behavior. We postulate that rapid and frequent administration of the drug interferes with the processes involved in terminating the activation of the orbitofrontal-thalamo-striatal circuit. This circuit which we postulate is initially activated by changes in dopamine, then deactivates as a function of time since last use of the drug. This deactivation does not occur in the abuser self-administering cocaine since its short half-life enables periodic administration that perpetuates the activation of the circuit without enab-ling its deactivation. For drugs with slow clearance kinetics at the dopa-mine transporter and for which the high decreases rapidly despite the presence of the drug in the brain, the rapid re-administration of the drug will be less effective in changing dopamine concentration (the first dose is still occupying the transporters) and hence in reactivating the circuit until eventually the circuit deactivates.[17] Though this discussion focuses on the relation between the kinetics of the drug at the dopamine transporter and its ability to induce continuous craving that is not satiated, it is also likely that environmental factors also contribute to the intake of the drug and by themselves may also initiate a craving reaction.[4,28]

The question then remains as to the mechanisms that account for this pathological activation of the orbitofrontal-thalamo-striatal circuit and its relation to enhanced dopaminergic activity induced by the drug. Percep-tion of pleasure is likely to underlie behaviors that need to be repeated in order for species survival.[29] Pleasure is used as a natural reinforcer to increase the probability of the animal engaging in a given behavior and maintaining that behavior once it has initiated it.[28] Thus the perception of pleasure which gives the stimuli it motivational properties has been associated with increased dopamine activity in the nucleus accumbens and may serve as a trigger for the maintenance of the behavior.[30] For physio-logical stimuli such as eating, drinking, or sex, the incentive motivational properties of the stimuli which appear to involve dopaminergic neurotransmission are followed by the consummatory response which is terminated by what humans subjectively describe as satiety. The consummatory component of the behavior is likely to involve the activation of neurotransmitters other than dopamine such as central opiates[28] as well as activation of frontal cortical areas since these are uniquely activated with reinforcer dependent stimulation and not with reinforcement independent stimulation.[31] Though the mechanisms underlying the termination of the consummatory component of the behavior (perception of satiety) are not well understood it is likely that they involve participation of the orbitofrontal cortex since its destruction can lead to the emergence of repetitive behaviors that cannot be terminated.[32] Dopaminergic regulation is also likely to play a role since a similar syndrome can be generated by the destruction of the mesocortical dopamine pathway.[33] Serotonergic neurotransmission is probably also involved since destruction of the serotonergic system increases the "drive" to self-administer the drug while enhancement of serotonergic activity significantly reduces it.[34,35] In humans pathology in the orbitofrontal cortex, cingulate gyrus and in the striatum has been linked with obsessive compulsive disorders[36,37] which share with addiction the compulsive quality of the behavior.[4] In fact acute intoxication with psychostimulants induces stereotypical behaviors in the user[38] and exacerbates compulsive symptomatology in patients with obsessive compulsive disorder,[39,40] indicating that both of these types of pathology may involve a common cerebral circuit.

Interestingly, in our studies with cocaine abusers dopamine D_2 receptor availability was found to be correlated with metabolic activity in the orbitofrontal cortex and cingulate gyrus suggesting an association between dopamine activity and function of these cortical brain regions. This association could reflect either a modulation by dopamine of these brain regions[41] or alternatively it could represent modulation of dopamine activity by frontal-striatal circuits.[31,42] Assuming that changes occurring in the nigro-striatal dopamine pathway (which are the ones measures with PET and D_2 receptor ligands) are similar to those in the meso-cortical dopamine pathway one could interpret the correlation as reflecting dopaminergic activity from the ventral tegmental area modulating activity in the orbitofrontal cortex and cingulate gyrus.[35,43] However, this relation could also occur indirectly via the striato-pallido-thalamic-cortical circuit.[44,45] In this model increased dopaminergic activation would change activity in these two frontal regions and the rapid and repeated administration of cocaine would trigger a continuous state of hyperactivity perceived as intense desire for the drug, loss of control and failure to terminate the use of the drug. This state would take over the behavior of the subject perpetuating drug self-administration despite tolerance to the pleasurable effects of cocaine.[46] In this respect it is interesting to note that experiments in animals have shown that both the orbitofrontal cortex as well as the medial prefrontal cortex can initiate neuronal activity in circuits that mediate reinforcement.[47]

This still leaves the question unanswered of what are the mechanisms that account for the differences in responses observed between the cocaine addict and the non-addict. Our study shows abnormalities in metabolic activity in the orbitofrontal cortex and cingulate gyrus both during early[9] and late cocaine withdrawal,[10] which change from hypermetabolic to hypometabolic. The direct association between metabolic activity in these brain regions and dopamine D_2 receptors[13] indicates that manipulation of dopaminergic circuits may activate or deactivate these brain regions. We believe that cocaine activates these cortical regions by increasing dopamine activity in meso-cortical as well as meso-striatal pathways and that this activation is maintained by its frequent administration. We also postulate that the threshold for activation of this circuit lowers as a function of chronic cocaine exposure and that this is likely to involve changes in receptor-effector signaling mechanisms that initiate the behavior even after small changes in dopamine release as may occur for example when addicts are exposed to drug paraphernalia. With protracted withdrawal the reduction in dopamine D_2 receptors remains but without the use of cocaine there is no longer dopaminergic activation of the orbitofrontal circuit which becomes hypometabolic. However, in these subjects the threshold for activation remains low such that if exposed to stimuli that raise dopamine levels, i.e., stress,[46] alcohol,[49] small doses of cocaine and/or memories associated with cocaine, the orbitofrontal-striatal circuit is activated generating the drive and loss of control for consuming cocaine. However, it is also possible that the abnormalities occur at the level of the orbitofrontal cortex and/or cingulate gyrus which then becomes hyper-responsive to dopaminergic stimulation and hyporesponsive to deactivating signals that would normally terminate the behaviors. Dysfunction of the orbitofrontal cortex and/or cingulate gyrus could result, among others, from changes in dopaminergic as well as serotonergic neurotransmission.

In summary, based on results from our PET studies we postulate that cocaine addiction results from the frequent repeated stimulation of meso-cortical and meso-striatal dopaminergic pathways which activates the orbitofrontal-thalamo-striatal circuit that then serves to perpetuate its continuous and repeated administration after tolerance to the pleasurable effects of the drug have occurred and even in the presence of negative side effects.

From this perspective, the pleasurable properties of cocaine serve as a trigger for the activation of a circuit that will then maintain the consummatory behavior. Lower threshold for activation and higher threshold for deactivation of this circuit may be one of the mechanisms accounting for the loss of control and the compulsive drug intake in the addicted individual.

REFERENCES

1. Johanson CE, Fishman MW. The pharmacology of cocaine related to its abuse. Pharmacol Rev 1989; 41:3-52.

2. Koob GF, Bloom FE. Cellular and molecular mechanisms of drug dependence. Science 1988; 242:715-723.

3. Gawin FH. Cocaine addiction: psychology and neurophysiology. Science 1991; 151:1580-1586.

4. Robinson TE, Berridge KC. The neural basis of drug craving: an incentive-sensitization theory of addiction. Brain Research Reviews 1993; 18:247-291.

5. Modell JG, Mounts JM, Curtis G, Greden J. Neurophysiologic dysfunction in basal ganglia/limbic striatal and thalamocortical circuits as a pathogenetic mechanism of obsessive compulsive disorder. J Neuropsych 1989; 1:27-35.

6. Fowler JS, Wolf AP, Volkow ND. New directions in positron emission tomography. In: Bristol JA. ed. Annual Reports in Medicinal Chemistry. San Diego; Academic Press, 1990:261-269.

7. London ED, Cascella NG, Wong DF, Phillips RL, Sannals RF, Links JM, Herning R, Grayson R, Jaffe JH. Cocaine-induced reduction of glucose utilization in human brain. A study using positron emission tomography and [fluorine-18]-fluorodeoxyglucose. Arch General Psychiatry 1990; 47:567-574.

8. Volkow ND, Mullani N, Gould L, Krajewski K, Adler S. Cerebral blood flow in chronic cocaine users. Brit J Psychiatry 1988; 152:641-648.

9. Volkow ND, Fowler JS, Wolf AP, Hitzemann R, Dewey S, Bendriem B, Alpert R, Hoff A. Changes in brain glucose metabolism in cocaine dependence and withdrawal. Am J Psych 1991; 148:621-626.

10. Volkow ND, Hitzemann R, Wag GJ, Fowler JS, Wolf AP, Dewey SL. Long-term frontal brain metabolic changes in cocaine abusers. Synapse 1992; 11:184-190.

11. Baxter LR, Schwartz JM, Phelps M, Mazziotta JC, Barrio J, Rawson RA, Engel J, Guze BH, Selin C, Sumida R. Localization of neurochemical effects of cocaine and other stimulants in the human brain. J Clin Psychiatry 1988; 4:923-926.

12. Volkow ND, Fowler J, Wolf A, Schlyer D, Shiue Ch, Albert R, Dewey S, Logan J, Bendriem B, Christman D, Hitzemann R, Henn F. Effects of chronic cocaine abuse on postsynaptic dopamine receptors. Am J Psychiatry 1990; 147:719-724.

13. Volkow ND, Fowler JS, Wang G-J, Hitzemann R, Logan J, Schlyer D, Dewey S, Wolf AP. Dopaminergic dysregulation of frontal metabolism may contribute to cocaine addiction. Synapse 1993; 14:169-177.

14. Fowler JS, Volkow ND, Wolf AP, Dewey SL, Schlyer DJ, MacGregor R, Hitzemann R, Logan J, Bendriem B, Christman D. Mapping cocaine-binding sites in human and baboon brain *in vivo*. Synapse 1989; 4:371-377.

15. Fowler JS, Volkow ND, MacGregor RR, Logan J, Dewey SL, Galley SJ, Wolf AP. Comparative PET Studies of the kinetics and distribution of cocaine and cocaethylene in baboon brain. Synapse 1992; 12:220-227.

16. Fowler JS, Volkow ND, Logan J, MacGregor RR, Wang G-J, Wolf AP. Alcohol intoxication does not change cocaine pharmacokinetics in human brain and heart. Synapse 1992; 12:228-235.

17. Volkow ND, Ding Y-S, Fowler JS, Wang GJ, Logan J, Gatley JS, Dewey SL, Ashby C, Lieberman J, Hitzemann R, Wolf AP. Is methylphenidate like cocaine? Studies on their pharmacokinetics and distribution in human brain. Arch Gen Psychiatry 1995; 52:456-463. Copyright 1995, American Medical Association.

18. Volkow ND, Fowler JS, Wolf AP, Wang GJ, Logan J, MacGregor R, Dewey SL, Schlyer DJ, Hitzemann R. Distribution of ^{11}C-Cocaine in human heart, lungs, liver and adrenals. A dynamic PET study. J Nucl Med 1992; 33:521-525.

19. Ritz MC, Lamb RJ, Goldberg SR, Kuhar MJ. Cocaine receptors on dopamine transporters are related to self-administration of cocaine. Science 1987; 237:1219-1223.

20. Parran TV, Jasinski DR. Intravenous methylphenidate abuse: prototype for prescription drug abuse. Arch Intern Med 1991; 151:781-783.

21. Ding Y-S, Fowler JS, Volkow ND, Galley SJ, Logan J, Dewey S, Alexoff D, Wolf AP. Pharmacokinetics and *in vivo* Specificity of [11C]*dl-threo*-Methylphenidate for the Presynaptic Dopaminergic Neuron Synapse 1994; 18:152-160.

22. Cook CE, Jeffcoat AR, Perez-Reyes M. Pharmacokinetic studies of cocaine and phencyclidine in man. In: Barnett G, Chiang CN, eds. Pharmacokinetics and Pharmacodynamics of Psychoactive Drugs. Foster City, CA: Biomedical Publication, 1985:48-74.

23. Di Chiara G, Imperato A. Drugs abused by humans preferentially increase synaptic dopamine concentration in the mesolimbic system of freely moving rats. Proc Natl Acad Sci 1988; 85:5274-5278:

24. Modell JG, Mountz JM, Beresford TP. Basal ganglia/limbic striatal and thalamocortical involvement in craving and loss of control in alcoholism. Journal of Neuropsychiatry 1990; 2:123-144.

25. Bergman J, Madras B, Johnson SE, Spealman RD. Effects of cocaine and related drugs in nonhuman primates. III. Self administration by squirrel monkeys. J Pharmacol Exp Ther 1989; 251:150-155.

26. Johanson CE, Shuster CR. A choice procedure for drug reinforcers: cocaine and methylphenidate in the rhesus monkey. J Pharmacol Exper Ther 1975; 193:676-688.

27. Wilson MC, Hitomi M, Schuster CR. Psychomotor self administration as a function of dosage per injection in the rhesus monkey. Psychopharmacology 1971; 22:271-281.

28. Taylor JR, Robbins TW. Enhanced behavioral control by conditioned reinforcers following microinjections of d-amphetamine in the nucleus accumbens. Psychopharmacology 1984; 84:405-412.

29. Di Chiara G, Acquas E, Carboni E. Drug Motivation and abuse: a neurobiological perspective. In: Kalivas PW & Samson HH, eds. The Neurobiology of Drug and Alcohol Addiction. New York: Annals New York Academy of Sciences. 1992; 654:207-219.

30. Phillips AG, Pfaus JG, Blaha CD. Dopamine and motivated behavior: insights provided by in vivo analyses. In: Willner P & Scheel-Kruger J, eds. The Mesolimbic Dopamine System: From Motivation to Action. Chichester UK: John Wiley & Sons Ltd. 1991:199-224.

31. Porrino LJ, Esposito RU, Seeger TF, Crane AM, Pert A, Sokoloff L. Metabolic mapping of brain during rewarding self stimulation. Science 1984:224:306-309.

32. Kolb B. Studies on the caudate putamen and the dorsomedial thalamic nucleus: implications for mammalian frontal lobe function. Physiol Behav 1977; 18:237-244.

33. Le Moal M, Simon H. Mesocorticolimbic dopaminergic network: functional and regulatory notes. Physiol Rev 1991; 71:155-234.

34. Loh EA, Roberts DCS. Break points on a progressive ratio schedule reinforced by intravenous cocaine increases following depletion of forebrain serotonin. Psychopharmacology 1990; 101:262-266.

35. Richardson ER, Roberts CS. Fluoxetine pretreatment reduces breaking points on a progressive ratio schedule reinforced by intravenous self administration in the rat. Life Sciences 1991; 49:833-840.

36. Baxter LR, Phelps ME, Mazziotta J, Gum BH, Schwartz JM, Selin CE. Local cerebral glucose metabolic rates in obsessive compulsive disorder: a comparison with rates in unipolar depression and normal controls. Arch Gen Psych 1987; 44:211-218.

37. Insel TR. Towards a neuroanatomy of obsessive-compulsive disorder. Arch Gen Psychiatry 1992; 49:739-744.

38. Schiorring E. Psychopathology induced by "speed drugs." Pharmacol Biochem Behav. 1981; 1:109-122.

39. McDougle CJ, Goodman WK, Delgado PL, Price LH. Pathophysiology of obsessive-compulsive disorder. Am J Psychiatry 1989; 146:1350-1351.

40. Leonard HL, Rapoport JL. Relief of obsessive-compulsive symptoms by LSD and psilocin (letter). Am J Psychiatry 1987; 144:1239-1240.

41. Glowinski J, Tassin JP, Thierry Am. The mesocortical-prefrontal dopaminergic neurons. TINS 1984; Nov:415-418.

42. Selemon LD, Goldman-Rakic PS. Longitudinal topography and interdigitations of corticostriatal projections in the rhesus monkey. J Neurosci 1984; 5:776-794.

43. Stuss DT, Benson DF. The Frontal Lobes. New York: Raven Press, 1986.

44. Haber SN. Neurotransmitters in the human and nonhuman primate basal ganglia. Human Neurobiol 1986; 5:159-168.

45. Heimer L, Alheid GF, Zaborzky L. The basal ganglia. In: Paxinos G ed. The Rat Nervous System. Sidney: Academic Press, 1985:37-74.

46. Fischman MW, Schuster CR, Javaid J, Hatano Y, Davis J. Acute tolerance development to the cardiovascular and subjective effects of cocaine. J Pharmacol Exp Ther 1985; 235:677-682.

47. Dworkin SI, Smith JE. Cortical regulation of self administration. In: Kalivas PW & Samson HH, eds. The Neurobiology of Drug and Alcohol Addiction. New York: Annals New York Academy of Sciences. 1992; 654:274-281.

48. Abercrombie ED, Keefe HA, DiFrischia DS, Zigmond MJ. Differential effect of stress on in vivo dopamine release in striatum, nucleus accumbens, and medial prefrontal cortex. J Neurochem 1989; 52:1655-1658.

49. Gessa GL, Muntoni F, Collu M, Vargiu L, Mereu GP. Low doses of ethanol activate dopaminergic neurons in the ventral tegmental area. Brain Res 1985; 348:201-203.

Cocaine, Dopamine
and the Endogenous Opioid System

Mary Jeanne Kreek, MD

SUMMARY. Cocaine addiction and opiate addiction are both major health problems in the United States today. Prospective studies from our Laboratory, which were able to detect the advent of the HIV-1 epidemic in parenteral drug abusers in New York City beginning around 1978, also showed that, from the beginning of the AIDS epidemic, cocaine abuse was a very important co-factor significantly increasing the risk for developing cocaine dependency. Fundamental studies from many laboratories including our own have shown that cocaine has profound effects on dopaminergic function, primarily from its well-established primary action of blocking the reuptake of dopamine from the synaptic cleft, an action of cocaine directed at the specific dopamine transporter. It has also been well-established by others that cocaine similarly blocks the reuptake of serotonin and nor-

Mary Jeanne Kreek is Professor and Head, Laboratory of the Biology of Addictive Diseases, The Rockefeller University, New York, NY.

Address correspondence to: Mary Jeanne Kreek, MD, Box 171, The Rockefeller University, 1230 York Avenue, New York, NY 10021.

This work was conducted with support from a NIH-NIDA Research Center grant P50-DAO5130, a NIH-NIDA Research Scientific Award grant NIH-NIDA KO5-DA00049, a grant from the New York State Office of Alcoholism and Substance Abuse Services, a General Clinical Research Center grant (M01-RR00102) from the National Center for Research Resources at the National Institutes of Health, and also in part from the Aaron Diamond Foundation.

[Haworth co-indexing entry note]: "Cocaine, Dopamine and the Endogenous Opioid System." Kreek, Mary Jeanne. Co-published simultaneously in *Journal of Addictive Diseases* (The Haworth Medical Press, an imprint of The Haworth Press, Inc.) Vol. 15, No. 4, 1996, pp. 73-96; and: *The Neurobiology of Cocaine Addiction: From Bench to Bedside* (ed: Herman Joseph, and Barry Stimmel) The Haworth Medical Press, an imprint of The Haworth Press, Inc., 1996, pp. 73-96. Single or multiple copies of this article are available for a fee from The Haworth Document Delivery Service [1-800-342-9678, 9:00 a.m. - 5:00 p.m. (EST). E-mail address: getinfo@haworth.com].

epinephrine. However, recent studies from our laboratory have shown that chronic cocaine administration profoundly disrupts the endogenous opioid system. Extensive studies have been conducted using an animal model which we have developed in our laboratory, the "binge" pattern cocaine administration model. Findings from these studies have led us to recognize the profound disruption of both dynorphin gene expression and kappa opioid receptor gene expression in a setting of chronic cocaine administration and, in turn, have led us to question a possible role of disruption of this system in the acquisition and persistence of cocaine addiction. These findings may have significance for the development of new pharmacotherapeutic agents which may be directed to specific components of the endogenous opioid system and, in particular, possibly the kappa opioid receptor system. Therefore, we have initiated studies to examine further the role of the dynorphin peptide-kappa opioid receptor system in normal physiologic function in humans. *[Article copies available for a fee from The Haworth Document Delivery Service: 1-800-342-9678. E-mail address: getinfo@haworth.com]*

INTRODUCTION

Recent published household surveys have estimated that 24 million persons in the United States have used cocaine at some time. At least 600,000-700,000 are "hardcore" long-term addicts; it is estimated that at least two million have a disruption of function and are addiction-bound and/or already addicted to cocaine by most definitions. Recently it has been estimated that over 2.7 million persons have used heroin at some time; approximately one million of those meet the criteria of "hardcore" heroin dependency, defined as multiple daily uses, with the development of tolerance, physical dependence and drug-seeking behavior, and with the duration of abuse operationally defined (for purposes of the Federal guidelines governing access to methadone or LAAM maintenance treatment) as one year or more.[1-3] Co-morbidity is extraordinarily common between cocaine dependency and opiate dependency. Over 80% of "hardcore" heroin addicts seeking treatment in the New York City area are also now cocaine abusers or cocaine dependent.[1,4-6] There is an even greater problem of co-morbidity of both cocaine and heroin addiction with alcohol and tobacco abuse; however, this paper will focus on cocaine dependency, cocaine dependency with co-morbidity of heroin dependency, and also the interactions of these drugs of abuse neurobiologically with the endogenous opioid and dopaminergic systems.

COCAINE, OPIATES AND HIV-1/INFECTION

AIDS awakened the world with respect to the magnitude of the drug abuse problem.[4,6-21] By unbanking blood which had been banked prospectively in my Laboratory at the Rockefeller University from 1969 onward, and using the first available reliable assays for HIV-1 antibody developed, working in collaboration with the CDC, in 1983-84, we were able to define when the HIV-1 infection entered the New York City parenteral drug-abusing, primarily heroin-addicted population.[7,8,10] We found that parenteral drug abusers in New York City first were infected with the AIDS virus around 1978, and that the prevalence of infection with HIV rapidly rose until 1983 when a plateau was reached, with around 50-60% of parenteral drug abusers not in treatment for their primary addiction to opiates infected with the HIV-1.[7,8,10,14] We also found that the great preponderance of those who became infected with HIV-1 early on were already co-dependent with cocaine.[4] Thus, concomitant cocaine abuse and intravenous heroin addiction was a major vulnerability factor for getting HIV-1 infection in the early days of the epidemic.[4,7,8,10]

We also learned in 1983-84 that of those persons who had been fortunate enough to enter an effective methadone maintenance treatment program before 1978, when the AIDS epidemic hit New York City, and who stayed in treatment, less than 10% were HIV-1 infected in 1984, a time when over 50% of untreated street addicts were infected.[7,8,10] These findings have been replicated in Sweden by Blix and elsewhere.[11] Similar findings have been made subsequently by many groups in the United States; there is no doubt that effective methadone maintenance treatment, with use of proper doses and proper adjunctive services, can be a very strong protector against HIV-1 infection, as well as other infectious diseases.[6-21] These findings underscore the urgent need for us to continue our search for an effective pharmacotherapy for cocaine dependency, and to combine such pharmacotherapy with behavioral treatments, which will continue to be important as adjunctive treatments when used along with pharmacotherapy of cocaine addiction. However, behavioral treatment alone has not been able to achieve the levels of long-term success that one needs to achieve, just as behaviorally-based drug-free approaches when used alone have not been able to achieve a significant level of success in heroin addicts with long-term addiction. Specific pharmacotherapy for opiate addiction, primarily using the long-acting opioid, methadone, in long-term maintenance treatment, or now alternatively, l-alpha-acetylmethadol (LAAM) treatment, combined with effective behavioral treatments, can provide high levels of success.[1-3,6,22-27]

NEUROBIOLOGICAL BASIS OF ADDICTIVE DISEASES

We have hypothesized, for many years, that addictive diseases–and we consider them specific addictive diseases: opiate dependency, stimulant dependency, and alcoholism, with some overlap, but each with some independent and specific individual features–may be due to a variety of factors, including genetic predisposition in some persons, drug induced abnormalities in many or all persons, and specific host response and environmental factors in most who become addicted.[1,3,22-27]

POSSIBLE GENETIC FACTORS IN ADDICTIVE DISEASES

First, we have hypothesized that in some persons, there may be genetic factors.[1-3] My Laboratory has an established collaboration with Dr. Lei Yu of the University of Indiana; our first studies of the possible molecular genetics of opioid dependency in humans involved exploring the variability, or heterogeneity of alleles, in various defined populations of persons without and with addictive diseases, of the human mu opiate receptor recently cloned by the groups of Yu and others. We have hypothesized that any genetic factors involved in specific addictions will not be due to a single gene, but rather to multiple genes; therefore, our group and others will explore the possible role of many genes. Undoubtedly, any genetic variability contributing to the development of addictions will turn out to be multi-factorial making scientific explorations difficult; yet, we will at-. tempt to pursue these molecular genetic studies carefully, as will many other research groups throughout the world.

DRUG-INDUCED ALTERATIONS IN NORMAL PHYSIOLOGY

Secondly, and no longer a hypothesis, we know the drugs of abuse, including opiates and also cocaine, effect alterations of normal physiology, and these alterations may be persistent and/or permanent.[1,3,22-27] Also, these changes may, in part, contribute to drug craving or "hunger," and thus to relapse to drug use. Such drug-induced alterations in physiology should continue to be studied, both in animal models and in human subjects as appropriate, to determine where we should target pharmacotherapeutic agents, that is, at specific sites of action, receptors, or neurochemical systems, that may be deranged by drug abuse, with the goal of normalization of functions.

ROLE OF STRESSORS AND "SET AND SETTING" IN ADDICTIVE DISEASES

Finally, we know that there are variable host responses to drugs of abuse.[1-3] Vulnerable persons may be unmasked by use of potentially addicting drugs, but a variety of factors may modulate individual initial and continuing responses to drug abuse, ranging from "set and setting," environmental conditions, presence of other diseases, which may alter the response to drugs, and age and developmental status. Our Laboratory, for over twenty years, has hypothesized that an atypical responsivity to stress and stressors may contribute either to the unmasking of what may be an inherent predisposition, and/or may be a central component of drug-induced changes, conferring vulnerability to develop addiction, and also that such atypical responsivity to stress may contribute to the persistence of, and relapse to, drug abuse.[1,3,22-27]

THE ENDOGENOUS OPIOID SYSTEM

We have asked the question of what may be the role of the endogenous opioid system in three addictive diseases under study in my Laboratory: heroin addiction, cocaine dependency and alcoholism. There is increasing evidence from our Laboratory and others that the endogenous opioid system may be deranged not only in heroin addiction, in which such alterations might be anticipated, since exogenous opiates like the endogenous opioids bind to the specific opioid receptors, but also in cocaine dependency and alcoholism.

OPIOID RECEPTORS

Based on very early hypotheses of Dole and others, several early studies were performed by Dole, Goldstein and others to attempt to document the existence of specific opiate receptors.[28,29,30] However, the specific activity of the radioactivity labeled, stereoselective opioid receptor ligands was too low to allow elucidation of stereoselective specific opioid receptors.[28-30] Three years later, with the availability of high specific activity radiolabeled naloxone and etorphine, three groups, within a short interval of time, were able to simultaneously define and report the existence of specific opiate receptors.[31,32,33] Snyder, Simon and Terenius, working independently and with different radiolabeled ligands, defined the fact that there are specific stereoselective binding sites for opiates.[31,32,33] Over the next twenty years, it was defined that there were at least three types of opioid receptors. This was achieved by studying the binding of specifically synthesized synthetic chemical ligands with increasing selectivity for binding at these receptor sites types: mu, delta and kappa. Some research suggested that there were subtypes to each of these, and in fact, the synthetic chemical ligand research work still suggests the existence of receptor subtypes.

Molecular biologists trying to clone these receptors were not successful until late 1992, when again simultaneously, but independently, and using similar techniques of expression cloning, Kieffer in Strasbourg, France and Evans working at UCLA in California were able to clone, from a rodent/hybrid cell line, the delta opioid receptor.[34,35] This was soon followed by the cloning of the mu opioid receptor, by both Yu in Indiana and Uhl of the intramural program of National Institute on Drug Abuse,[36,37] followed soon by cloning of the kappa opioid receptor by Yu.[38] Within one to six months, several other groups had succeeded in cloning each of these different opioid receptors and reported their findings. There has been also an "orphan" opioid-like receptor cloned which was found not to bind with affinity of specificity with any exogenous or endogenous opioid.

There is extensive homology in the amino acid sequence of each of the types of specific opioid receptors, especially in the seven transmembrane regions that transverse the cell membrane. The differences are primarily outside the cell in the N-terminus, as well as in some of the extracellular loops. Also within the cell, at the carboxyl terminus and in some of the intracellular loops, where signal transduction occurs, there are some distinct differences. The homology from man to mouse and rat also is very high.

OPIOID PEPTIDES

There are three classes of endogenous opioid peptides; each class is derived from a single gene with a single large peptide initially produced: (1) endorphins–one gene, one product, proopiomelanocortin, is extremely exciting because it yields equimolar amounts of beta endorphin and ACTH, the well-known mammalian stress responsive neuropeptide; (2) enkephalins–one gene, one product, proenkephalin, yielding multiple opioid peptides; and (3) dynorphins–one gene, one product, prodynorphin, which yields a variety of both opioid and also biologically active non-opioid neuropeptides. The question therefore can be addressed as what may be the role of these three classes of endogenous opioid peptides, which bind in overlapping selectivity to the three types of specific opioid receptors, in each of the addictive diseases?

The endogenous ligand for the "orphan" opioid receptor remained unknown when this paper was presented. However, in the late autumn of 1995, two independent groups in France and in Switzerland discovered and defined a novel ligand "nociceptin" or "orphanin" for this orphan opioid receptor.[39,40] Although the search for other specific subtypes of opioid receptors is still going on, no group has cloned subtypes of mu, delta or kappa receptors.

DOPAMINE AND THE BRAIN
"PLEASURE" OR "REWARD" CENTER

The reinforcing effects of drugs of abuse, the so-called "pleasurable" or "rewarding" effects, have been defined and studied by many groups and seem to be related in large part to the dopaminergic systems, especially the mesolimbic-mesocortical dopaminergic system, with dopaminergic cell bodies in the ventral tegmental area with projections to the nucleus accumbens, the so-called "pleasure" or "reward" center, as well as to other regions of the mesolimbic-mesocortical dopaminergic system, such as the amygdala, olfactory tubercles and the cingulate cortex. There are also dopaminergic neurons in the substantia nigra with projections releasing dopamine in the caudate putamen part of the striatum, a known site of the locomotor activity effects of drugs of abuse. These acute effects, which are "pleasurable" or "rewarding," seem to be related directly to the "reinforcing" effects of drugs of abuse which lead to the self-administration of the addicting drugs by animal models or humans. In addition, and either completely separate, or more likely connected in some ways, is the long-lasting "craving" or "drug hunger." This leads to perpetuation of, or relapse to, drug self-administration. Therefore, much of the research of our Laboratory has been focused on elucidating both the acute, but also persistent, neurochemical and molecular events which underlie the reinforcing properties of drugs of abuse and which may lead to an understanding of the mechanisms of persistent "drug hunger" or "craving."

QUANTITATIVE MOLECULAR BIOLOGICAL STUDIES
OF THE ENDOGENOUS OPIOID SYSTEM

Our Laboratory using primarily the technique of solution hybridization protection assay, as modified in our NIDA Research Center, and others using a variety of techniques, have studied the distribution of the endogenous opioid system components in the rodent brain. We have found that several of the components are abundant in the same regions where dopa-minergic terminals are abundant, and which also have been documented to be involved in effects of drugs of abuse, that is, the mesolimbic-mesocorti-cal and nigrostriatal dopaminergic systems. We have hypothesized that mu and kappa opioid receptors (and possibly also the delta receptor) may be involved in the effects of each of the drugs of abuse).[41] We have also hypothesized that dynorphin itself, one of the endogenous opioid peptides acting at kappa opioid receptors, may act as a "brake" either distantly, for instance in the substantia nigra, or possibly also locally in the caudate putamen and also in the nucleus accumbens to alter dopaminergic tone.[41]

ALTERATIONS IN RNA LEVELS OR GENE EXPRESSION: IMPLICATIONS FOR ADDICTIONS

In my Laboratory and Center supported by National Institute on Drug Abuse primarily, several investigators, including Branch and colleagues, have developed a modified solution hybridization RNase protection assay which allows us now to measure quantitatively small amounts of gene messages (mRNA) of interest in a single brain region of a single ani-mal.[41-50] In this quantitative technique, very similar to analytical chemis-try, standard calibration curves are constructed for both the internal stan-dard (for which we usually use ribosomal 18s RNA), as well as for mRNAs of genes of interest.[41-50] Trichloracetic acid precipitation is used to harvest hybridized species, and radioactivity in hybridized species is determined after establishing that a single or predominant hybridized spe-cies is formed.[42]

Using these techniques, we are able to study quantitatively the levels of message of genes in individual brain regions of individual rats or mice. Using probes generously provided to us by the several groups who origi-nally cloned each gene of interest, we have, when needed, subcloned these cDNA probes to produce very large riboprobes, allowing us to have a stringent and also sensitive system to study the endogenous opioid system and related neuropeptides or neurotransmitter systems.[42] Using these tech-niques, we have found that the nucleus accumbens and caudate putamen region, known sites of actions of drugs of abuse, are very rich both in the mu and kappa opioid receptor gene expression.[41,43,44] Also abundant lev-els of mRNAs of the mu and kappa opioid receptor were found within the hypothalamus, possibly the brain's center for regulation of stress respon-sivity.[43,44] The levels of proenkephalin mRNA and prodynorphin mRNA were also very high in these important regions.[42,44-46]

STRESS HYPOTHESIS:
POSSIBLE NEUROBIOLOGICAL BASIS OF ADDICTIONS

Because of our early hypothesis that atypical responsivity to stress and stressors may contribute to the persistence of, and relapse to, addictive drug use and also possibly to the initial acquisition of addiction, we also are very interested in the distribution of the endogenous opioid system gene expression in the hypothalamus and pituitary as part of our studies of the role of the endogenous opioid system in modulation of this stress responsive, hypothalamic pituitary (adrenal) axis.[1,3,22-27,43,44,47-50] We have found using our modified quantitative technique that the levels of proenkephalin and prodynorphin mRNAs are also very high in these important regions.[41,42,44]

HYPOTHALAMIC-PITUITARY-ADRENAL AXIS ACTIVITY
IN SPECIFIC ADDICTIONS

In humans, both ACTH and beta endorphin are processed from proopiomelanocortin in the anterior-pituitary and circulate peripherally, effecting a variety of actions, including the well-established effect of ACTH in driving the adrenal cortex in man to synthesize and release the glucocorticoid, cortisol and in the rat or mouse, corticosterone. These glucocorticoids act in a negative feedback mode both at the hypothalamus and at the anterior pituitary to inhibit release of CRF and POMC peptides respectively. By acting in this negative feedback mode to reduce the release of CRF and POMC peptides, including the two stress responsive neuropeptides, beta endorphin and ACTH, temporarily sythesis and release of glucocorticoid by the adrenal is decreased and the negative feedback is then reduced. This results in a normal circadian rhythm of each of these hormones, that is, a daily rhythm with highest amounts of peripherally circulating peptides and steroids in the early morning and lower amounts towards evening in humans, and the converse in rodents which are primarily nocturnal in their activities.

RELATIONSHIP OF STRESS RESPONSIVE AXIS,
THE ENDOGENOUS OPIOIDS AND ADDICTION

Studies in Rodent Models

Using a rodent model, and large subcloned probes for both CRH and POMC genes, our Laboratory has confirmed and extended earlier studies from several other laboratories of the brain distribution of these genes, and has quantitatively measured the levels of their expression.[47-50] In addition to substantial levels of CRF in the hypothalamus and frontal cortex, as well as in the brain stem, we have confirmed that CRF mRNA is found in measurable amounts in an important region of the mesolimbic-mesocortical dopaminergic system, the amygdala, which is possibly involved in emotional responses. Similarly, our Laboratory has found that POMC mRNA is present in measurable amounts in the amygdala, as well as in the pituitary and hypothalamus.[47-50] However, when we asked the question of whether glucocorticoid, in this case, the synthetic glucocorticoid dexamethasone, could exert its negative feedback at each of these sites, we found, as had a few previously reported studies from other laboratories using different techniques, primarily *in situ* hybridization, that dexamethasone would act exclusively in the hypothalamus, that is the site of HPA axis regulation.[47-50]

Studies in Humans

We have also conducted extensive neuroendocrine studies in humans, both healthy volunteers and volunteers with defined addictive diseases.[1,3,51] We now know from the work of many laboratories, including Fischmann, Sarnyai, Rivier, Mendelson and Mello and others, including my own, that acutely, and also during chronic administration in animal models and in man, cocaine will cause an enhanced release of glucocorticoid, presumably due to increased release of CRF and, in turn, ACTH and beta endorphin, just as happens after administration of alcohol or of an opioid antagonist, or in the setting of withdrawal of a "hardcore" heroin addict from opiates.[48,51-56] Conversely, in humans, short-acting opiates, such as heroin or morphine, both acutely and chronically suppress release of ACTH and in turn suppress cortisol release, and create abnormalities, usually a flattening, of the normal circadian rhythm of levels of these hormones.[1-3,21-27,51,57-66] Cocaine has been reported by different investigators to both enhance and decrease serum prolactin levels in humans; this is probably primarily due to when the cocaine-dependent person was studied with respect to their last exposure to cocaine. Opiates acutely, and when administered on a chronic basis in both rodent models and in humans, cause release of prolactin.[57,66]

We have also studied the effects of metyrapone, a compound which blocks the last step of cortisol synthesis in man, at the adrenal cortex level.[1,3,6,21-26,56,58,60,62,64-66] By blocking cortisol synthesis, there is a prompt reduction in the usual negative feedback controlled by cortisol of CRF and POMC peptide synthesis and release; therefore, one expects to see normally a two- to four-fold increase in plasma levels of circulating ACTH and beta endorphin. We have found that in long-term, stabilized, methadone maintained patients, with no ongoing drug or alcohol abuse, normal basal levels of ACTH, beta endorphin, and cortisol are achieved along with normal circadian rhythm thereof; there is also a normal response to this chemically-induced stressor that is, metyrapone.[1,3,6,21-27,51,57,59,61,63,65,66]

ATYPICAL STRESS RESPONSIVITY IN SPECIFIC ADDICTIVE DISEASES

In contrast, there is a hyporesponsivity to this chemically-induced stress in active heroin addicts; very provocatively, in drug-free former heroin addicts, there is an atypically hyperresponsive state.[1,3,51,61,63,66] Such hyperresponsivity, of which we made a preliminary report in 1984 based on our early findings, previously had not been detected in any neuroendocrine studies in humans.[61] Very recently, we have also found a similar hyperresponsivity in pilot studies conducted among recently abstinent cocaine-dependent persons.[1,3,51] These findings have led us to ask very specifically about the interactions of the stress-responsive axis, which includes at least one endogenous opioid, beta endorphin, and other aspects of the endogenous opioid system, including mu and possibly also kappa type opioid receptors, along with the dopaminergic system. We know that addicts on the street may use cocaine plus heroin together, the so-called "speedball," to get an atypical "high" or euphoric response.[1] But far more common is a second combination of cocaine and heroin use, that is, people who have begun their drug abuse history using cocaine, and then will begin to use heroin to self-medicate the "crash," and go on to develop heroin dependency and addiction with or without continuing cocaine dependency.[1,4,51,67]

EFFECTS OF COCAINE ON NEUROTRANSMITTERS AND NEUROPEPTIDES

We know from neurobiological studies of many research groups that the primary action of cocaine is very specifically and primarily to block the binding of dopamine to the dopamine transporter and thereby to prevent the reuptake from the synapse into the presynaptic neuronal endings. In addition, and to a lesser extent, cocaine blocks the reuptake of serotonin and norepinephrine from the synapse by their respective specific transporters. Cocaine, unlike amphetamines, does not cause release of dopamine, but rather blocks its reuptake, thus increasing the extracellular fluid and synaptic concentrations of this neurotransmitter. This accumulation of dopamine in the synapse may cause increased activity by dopamine at D_1, D_2, and any other specific dopamine receptors located at the post-synaptic site in the brain regions of interest, as well as at least one dopamine auto-receptor at the pre-synaptic sites. From the recent studies of our Laboratory, using our "binge" pattern cocaine administration model, we have learned that the endogenous opioid system is also profoundly disrupted by chronic cocaine administration.

"BINGE" PATTERN COCAINE ADMINISTRATION: ANIMAL MODEL OF A HUMAN ADDICTIVE DISEASE

In my Laboratory, we have modeled the "binge" pattern of cocaine administration in rodents from the most common pattern of abuse in humans, which we know well from our patient populations.[1,3-6,41-46,48,67-76] Using this experimental design, modeled after the most common pattern of human abuse of cocaine, and which was developed by my Laboratory starting in 1988, we have conducted several related studies.[41-46,48,67-76] Animals are given three doses of cocaine (5 to 20 mg/kg each), one hour apart, with no cocaine then for 22 hours; a variety of behavioral, neurochemical and molecular measurements are made. Cocaine is administered just before what would be the sleep period for the rat, that is, in the early morning hours. Dr. E. Unterwald and Dr. A. Ho and other colleagues in my Laboratory using this paradigm, have conducted studies characterizing the pattern of behavior effected on the first day of this "binge" pattern cocaine administration.[73] Increased locomotor activity was observed after each of the three doses of cocaine.[73] After 13 days of daily "binge" pattern cocaine administration, we observed the well-documented (but usually following a protracted period of abstinence after repeated cocaine exposures) behavioral modification of "sensitization" to the locomotor effect of cocaine first described many years ago; and in our studies, we quantitated this sensitization by continuously monitoring in home cages to measure locomotor activity behavior.[73] It was found that there is enhanced activity after 13 days compared with day one of "binge" pattern cocaine administration.[73]

EFFECTS OF "BINGE" PATTERN COCAINE ADMINISTRATION ON DOPAMINE, DOPAMINE-RECEPTOR TRANSPORTER AND DOPAMINE RECEPTORS

In parallel studies, Dr. I. Maisonneuve in my Laboratory, using the technique of microdialysis in awake, freely-moving rats, has shown that each dose of cocaine administered in the "binge" pattern on an acute basis causes increased dopamine concentrations in the extracellular fluid of the nucleus accumbens (the ventromedial striatum) and in the caudate putamen (the dorsolateral striatum).[71] Cocaine levels were measured also in the extracellular fluid of caudate putamen regions.[71] We were able to determine that the half-life of cocaine in this region, after the last injection of cocaine, is 37 minutes.[71] With the once an hour administration of cocaine in the "binge" pattern paradigm, an accumulation of cocaine occurs in the brain regions of interest. However, we found a flattening of levels of extracellular fluid dopamine concentrations after the first injection of cocaine, showing a relative "acute tolerance" or "adaptation" during this acute "binge" pattern cocaine administration.[71]

We also found that after 14 days of "binge" pattern cocaine administration, the resting basal levels of dopamine, measured in actual molar concentrations, in the extracellular fluid, are significantly reduced, in both the nucleus accumbens and the caudate putamen.[74] Although there is a steep rise in dopamine levels in the extracellular fluid, after each of three doses of cocaine, the actual measured levels achieved are never as great in the animals receiving "binge" pattern cocaine for the 14th day, as compared with animals pretreated with saline and receiving cocaine for the first time. If, on the other hand, the data are expressed as percent of baseline levels, the excursion or amplitudes of rise in dopamine levels in the extracellular fluid are as great, or even greater, in the nucleus accumbens and as great in the caudate putamen of the chronic cocaine treated animals.[74]

Dr. R. Spangler and C. Maggos in my Laboratory have asked the question of whether the dopamine transporter gene expression is altered in this setting of "binge" pattern cocaine administration.[75,76] At the end of the 14th day of "binge" pattern cocaine administration, they found no changes in levels of the message for the gene.[73-76] Other research groups have reported no change in binding by the dopamine transporter after chronic cocaine administration using different treatment protocols. However, there may be changes of significance in gene expression in the cocaine-free or abstinent period after chronic cocaine administration; further studies are in progress to address this question on a molecular basis.[75-76]

Dr. E. Unterwald in my Laboratory has asked the question of whether "binge" pattern cocaine administration alters binding of specific, selective ligands to the D_2 dopaminergic receptor, and has found that there are increases in binding in specific brain regions, including in the rostral caudate putamen, nucleus accumbens, and olfactory tubercle at the end of 7 days of "binge" pattern cocaine administration.[71] When animals were treated for 14 days, the D_2 receptors showed normal levels of binding the selective ligand.[73] In contrast, D_1 type dopaminergic receptor binding was found to be significantly increased at the end of 14 days of "binge" pattern cocaine administration and again in brain regions of interest with respect to the behavioral effects of drugs of abuse, the nucleus accumbens and another part of the mesolimbic-mesocorticol dopaminergic system, the olfactory tubercle.[73] These findings are especially provocative since the D_1 dopamine receptor has been linked with levels of dynorphin gene expression and of dynorphin peptide production.

EFFECTS OF "BINGE" PATTERN COCAINE ADMINISTRATION ON THE ENDOGENOUS OPIOID SYSTEM

Dr. E. Unterwald has also asked the question of what happens to specific opiate receptors in the setting of chronic pattern "binge" pattern cocaine administration in studies conducted in my Laboratory.[69,70,72] The binding of opioid receptors by specific receptor selective ligands after 14 days of "binge" pattern cocaine administration, as contrasted to controls which have received saline in the same pattern has been studied.[69,72] Significantly enhanced binding at mu opioid receptors was found in the caudate putamen, in the nucleus accumbens, in the cingulate gyrus and also in the basolateral amygdala, all regions with abundant dopaminergic terminals.[69,72] Kappa opioid receptor binding after "binge" pattern cocaine administration was also studied by Dr. Unterwald in my Laboratory; again, significant enhanced binding in similar brain regions was found, including in the caudate putamen, the nucleus accumbens, the cingulate cortex and also in the olfactory tubercles.[72] Thus, changes in both mu and kappa opioid receptor densities were identified in regions with abundant dopaminergic terminals, part of the mesolimbic-mesocortical and nigrostriatal dopaminergic systems. These are very provocative findings, suggesting increased activation, or ability to transmit signals by both the mu and kappa types of opioid receptors in these specific brain regions, in this setting of chronic "binge" pattern cocaine exposure. Other work has been performed or is in progress to look at the signal transduction mechanisms and other neurochemical and molecular events that may be associated with this enhanced density of mu and kappa opioid receptors.[70,77]

Drs. A. Branch and R. Spangler have studied what happens to the gene expression of specific classes of opioid peptide genes in this setting of chronic "binge" pattern cocaine administration.[42,45,46] Dr. Branch found no changes in levels of proenkephalin mRNA following 14 days of such treatment.[42] However, Dr. Spangler has found that after 14 days of "binge" pattern cocaine administration, and appearing first after 1 and 3 days of "binge" pattern cocaine administration, there is a significant and persistent upregulation of dynorphin gene expression, mRNA levels in the caudate putamen.[45,46] This increased prodynorphin gene expression is coupled with increased content of dynorphin peptides based on some preliminary work resulting from our collaboration with Dr. F. Nyberg of Uppsala, Sweden. All of these findings would suggest activation of the kappa opioid system, and also the mu opioid receptor system after "binge" pattern cocaine administration.

EXTRAPOLATION TO HUMANS: STUDIES OF THE ROLE OF THE DYNORPHIN PEPTIDE-KAPPA OPIOID RECEPTOR SYSTEM IN NORMAL PHYSIOLOGY AND IN ADDICTION

Therefore, we have initiated studies of the effects of dynorphin in humans.[78] These preliminary studies have been participated in by Drs. A. Ho, L. Borg, and in progress are more recent and ongoing studies participated in by Drs. J. Schluger, N. Bergasa, as well as Ms. M. Porter, Mr. S. Maniar, Mr. C. Maggos and Mr. M. Gunduz.[78] We have hypothesized that dynorphin A, by acting directly or indirectly to lower dopaminergic tone, which in humans is the primary modulator of prolactin release, may cause elevations in serum prolactin levels.[78] Dopaminergic tone provides tonic inhibition of prolactin release in humans through action in the tuberoinfundibular dopaminergic system, a different, but possibly parallel dopaminergic system to the mesolimbic-mesocortical and nigrostriatal systems.

With Dr. B. Chait who heads the Extended Range Mass Spectrometry Laboratory at The Rockefeller University, working in collaboration with Dr. J. Chou, and more recently, Dr. J. Yu, both chemists and mass spectrometrists in my Laboratory, we have been studying the processing of dynorphin peptides in humans, as well as in rats, *ex vivo* using techniques developed by Drs. Chou, Yu, Chait and colleagues.[79-84] Dynorphin A_{1-17}, the major natural endogenous kappa ligand and one of two initially processed peptides from prodynorphin, has 17 residues; Dynorphin A_{1-13}, a natural sequence but shortened dynorphin peptide is often used in neurobiological studies because it was the dynorphin peptide originally sequenced. Dynorphin A_{1-13} has been prepared for human use and made available (by N.T.I. Corporation, Richmond, CA) for use in our clinical research studies, along with dynoprhin A_{1-10} amide. We have conducted initial studies of the processing of this dynorphin A_{1-13} natural, but synthetic peptide, and find that it is very rapidly processed in human blood *ex vivo* to yield a major opioid product, dynorphin A_{1-12}, a minor opioid product, dynorphin A_{1-6} as well as several non-opioid products, primarily dynorphin A_{2-12} and $_{4-12}$.[79,81-83]

We have also conducted preliminary studies for this peptide in humans.[78] We administered this compound to normal human volunteers in a pilot study, which we reported recently and have found no response with respect to any changes in serum levels of prolactin occurred when placebo was administered, despite the fact that prolactin is a stress responsive hormone. However, when dynorphin A_{1-13} was administered intravenously, a prompt, dose-dependent rise in serum prolactin levels occurred, with a gradual decline over the next 120 minutes.[78] This preliminary study suggests that indeed dynorphin A_{1-13} acted at a specific hypothalamic site, altering (lowering) dopaminergic tone, resulting in enhanced prolactin release.[78] We now are asking the question of whether dynorphin, or a synthetic congener thereof, could be used to modulate dopaminergic tone in basal states, and whether such modulation and/or normalization of some of the disruptions seen in the setting of cocaine dependency would occur with use of such kappa receptor selective ligands.[78,80] This proposed modulation would be not unlike our strategy with methadone treatment, where we targeted the treatment agent towards a specific site of action.

COCAINE AND HEROIN ADDICTION: THE BENEFICIAL EFFECTS OF METHADONE MAINTENANCE

Dr. L. Borg in our laboratory has recently quantitated the prevalence of co-dependency of cocaine and heroin addiction.[5] Up to an 80% co-morbidity with cocaine dependency was found as the cocaine use "epidemic" increased.[1,4,5,6] However, with time in an effective methadone maintenance treatment program, with the intervals studied of 6 months, 53 months, and greater than 53 months, the percentage of all former heroin addicts remaining in methadone maintenance treatment (and with a high overall retention rate) who continued to use cocaine drugs dropped down to 30% and then on down to below 20%.[5]

We have always assumed that such reduction in the use of cocaine by long-term methadone maintenance patients in effective programs was because of the therapeutic milieu which is nurtured in any good methadone program. We still think that is the primary reason, but now with our findings concerning the disruption of the endogenous opioid system by chronic "binge" pattern cocaine exposure, we have to ask the question: Could there also be some pharmacological effectiveness of methadone in the reduction of cocaine use in co-dependent persons? Several groups have shown that buprenorphine, which is a partial mixed agonist/antagonist, but acts in humans primarily as a mu agonist, and also methadone and LAAM, both long-acting mu opioid receptor agonists, as well as morphine itself in rodent and subhuman primate models, will all decrease self-administration of cocaine. We now suggest that effective methadone programs not only provide a therapeutic milieu, but also may provide some pharmacological advantage in stabilizing the endogenous opioid system.

REFERENCES

1. Kreek MJ. Multiple drug abuse patterns and medical consequences. In: Meltzer HY, ed. Psychopharmacology: the third generation of progress. New York: Raven Press 1987:1597-1604.

2. Kreek MJ. Pharmacologic modalities of therapy: methadone maintenance and the use of narcotic antagonists. In: Stimmel B, ed. Heroin dependency: medical, economic and social aspects. New York: Stratton Intercontinental Medical Book Corp. 1975:232-290.

3. Kreek MJ. Rationale for maintenance pharmacotherapy of opiate dependence. In: O'Brien CP and Jaffe JH, eds. Addictive states New York: Raven Press, Ltd. 1992:205-230.

4. Novick DM, Trigg HL, Des Jarlais DC et al. Cocaine injection and ethnicity in parenteral drug users during the early years of the human immunodeficiency virus (HIV) epidemic in New York City. J Med Virol, 1989;:29:181-185.

5. Borg L, Broe DM, Ho A et al. Cocaine abuse is decreased with effective methadone maintenance treatment at an urban Department of Veterans Affairs (DVA) Program. In: Harris LS, ed. NIDA Research Monograph Series, Problems of Drug Dependence, 1994; Proceedings of the 56th Annual Scientific Meeting of the College on Problems of Drug Dependence. Rockville, MD: NIH Publication No. 95-3883, 1995:153:17.

6. Kreek MJ. Methadone maintenance treatment for harm reduction approach to heroin addiction. In: Loimer N, Schmid R, Springer A, eds. Drug addiction and AIDS. New York: Springer Verlag 1991:153-177.

7. Des Jarlais DC, Marmor M, Cohen H et al. Antibodies to a retrovirus etiologically associated with Acquired Immunodeficiency Syndrome (AIDS) in populations with increased incidences of the syndrome. Morbidity and Mortality Weekly Report 1984:33:377-379.

8. Novick D, Kreek MJ, Des Jarlais D et al. Antibody to LAV, the putative agent of AIDS, in parenteral drug abusers and methadone-maintained patients: abstract of clinical research findings: therapeutic, historical, and ethical aspects. In: Harris LS, ed. NIDA Research Monograph Series, Problems of Drug Dependence, 1985; Proceedings of the 47th Annual Scientific Meeting of The Committee on Problems of Drug Dependence. Rockville MD:DHHS Publication No. (ADM)86-1448, 1986:67:318-320.

9. Novick DM, Farci P, Karayiannis P, Gelb AM, Stenger RJ, Kreek MJ, Thomas HC. Hepatitis D virus antibody in HBsAg-positive and HBsAg-negative substance abusers with chronic liver disease. J Med Virol 1985:15:351-356.

10. Novick DM, Khan I, Kreek, MJ. Acquired immunodeficiency syndrome and infection with hepatitis viruses in individuals abusing drugs by injection. United Nations Bulletin on Narcotics. 1986:38:15-25.

11. Blix O. AIDS and IV heroin addicts: The preventative effect of methadone maintenance in Sweden. Proceedings of the 4th International Conference on AIDS, Stockholm, 1988:SR52.

12. Novick DM, Farci P, Croxson ST et al. Hepatitis delta virus and human immunodeficiency virus antibodies in parenteral drug abusers who are hepatitis B surface antigen positive. J Infect Dis. 1988:158:795-803.

13. Novick DM, Des Jarlais DC, Kreek MJ et al. The specificity of antibody tests for human immunodeficiency virus in alcohol and parenteral drug abusers with chronic liver disease. Alc Clin Exp Res. 1988:12:687-690.

14. Des Jarlais DC, Friedman SR, Novick DM et al. HIV-1 Infection among intravenous drug users in Manhattan, New York City 1977 to 1987. JAMA. 1989:261:1008-1012.

15. Kreek MJ. HIV-1 infection and parenteral drug abuse: ethical issues in diagnosis, treatment, research and the maintenance of confidentiality. In: Allebeck P, Jansson B, eds. Proceedings of the Third International Congress on Ethics in Medicine–Nobel Conference Series. New York: Raven Press, 1990:181-187.

16. Kreek MJ. Immune function in heroin addicts and former heroin addicts in treatment: pre/post AIDS epidemic. In: Pham PTK and Rice K, eds. Current chemical and pharmacological advances on drugs of abuse which alter immune function and their impact upon HIV-1 infection. Rockville, MD: NIDA Research Monograph Series, 1990:96:192-219.

17. Brown LS, Kreek MJ, Trepo C et al. Human immunodeficiency virus and viral hepatitis seroepidemiology in New York City intravenous drug abusers (IVDAs). In: Harris LS, ed. Problems of Drug Dependence, 1989; Proceedings of the 51st Annual Scientific Meeting of the Committee on Problems of Drug Dependence. Rockville, MD: NIDA Research Monograph Series DHHS Publication No. (ADM) 90-1663, 1990:95:443-444.

18. Kreek MJ, Des Jarlais DC, Trepo CL et al. Contrasting prevalence of delta hepatitis markers in parenteral drug abusers with and without AIDS. J Infect Dis. 1990; 162:538-541.

19. Kreek MJ. Pharmacological treatment of addiction: Normalization of physiology and AIDS risk reduction. In: Tagliamonte A and Maremmani I, eds. Drug Addiction and Related Clinical Problems. Wien, Germany: Springer-Verlag, 1995:165-173.

20. Borg L and Kreek MJ. Clinical problems associated with interactions between methadone pharmacotherapy and medications used in the treatment of HIV-positive and AIDS patients. Current Opinion in Psychiatry 1995; 8:199-202.

21. Kreek MJ. Biological correlates of methadone maintenance pharmacotherapy. In: Christoforov B, ed. Ann. Med. Interne: Intérêts et Limites des Traitements

de Substitution dans la Prise en Charge des Toxicomanes. Paris: Masson, 1994:145:9-14.

22. Kreek MJ. Medical safety, side effects and toxicity of methadone. Proceedings of the Fourth National Conference on Methadone Treatment. NAPAN-NIMH, 1972:171-174.

23. Kreek MJ. Medical safety and side effects of methadone in tolerant individuals. J Amer Med Assn. 1973: 223:665-668.

24. Kreek MJ. Physiological implications of methadone treatment. In: Methadone Treatment Manual. Washington, D.C.: U.S. Dept. of Justice (USGPO) #2700-00227, 1973:85-91.

25. Kreek MJ. Epilogue: Medical maintenance treatment for heroin addiction, from a retrospective and prospective viewpoint. In: State Methadone Maintenance Treatment Guidelines. Office for Treatment Improvement, Division for State Assistance, 1992:255-272.

26. Kreek MJ. The addict as a patient. In: Lowinson JH, Ruiz P, Millman RB and Langrod JG, eds. Substance Abuse: A Comprehensive Textbook. Baltimore, Maryland: Williams & Wilkins, 1992:997-1009.

27. Kreek MJ. Pharmacology and medical aspects of methadone treatment. In: Rettig RA and Yarmolinsky A, eds. Federal Regulation of Methadone Treatment. Washington, D.C.: National Academy of Sciences, National Academy Press, 1995:37-60.

28. Ingoglia NA and Dole VP. Localization of d- and l-methadone after intraventricular injection into rat brain. Journal of Pharmacology and Experimental Therapeutics. 1970: 175:84-87.

29. Dole VP, Biochemistry of addiction. Annual Review of Biochemistry. 1970:39:821-240.

30. Goldstein A, Lowney LT, Pal BK. Stereospecific and nonspecific interactions of the morphine congener levorphanol in subcellular fractions of mouse brain. Proceedings of the National Academy of Sciences of the United States of America, 1971:68:1742-1747.

31. Pert CB, Snyder SH. Opiate receptor: demonstration in nervous tissue. Science. 1973:179:1011-1014.

32. Simon EJ, Hiller JM, Edelman I. Stereospecific binding of the potent narcotic analgesic [3H]Etorphine to rat-brain homogenate. Proceedings of the National Academy of Sciences, 1973:70:1947-1949.

33. Terenius L. Stereospecific interaction between narcotic analgesics and a synaptic plasma membrane fraction of rat cerebral cortex. Acta Pharmacologica ET Toxicologica. 1973:32:317-320.

34. Evans CJ, Keith DE Jr., Morrison H, Magendzo, Edwards RH. Cloning of a delta opioid receptor by functional expression. Science. 1992:258:1952-1955.

35. Kieffer BL, Befort K, Gaveriaux-Ruff C, Hirth CG. The delto-opioid receptor: Isolation of a cDNA by expression cloning and pharmacological characterization. Proceedings of the National Academy of Science. 1992:89:12,048-12,052.

36. Chen Y, Mestek A, Liu J, Hurley JA, Yu L. Molecular cloning and functional expression of a mu opioid receptor from rat brain. Molecular Pharmacology. 1993:44:8-12.

37. Wang JB, Imai Y, Eppler CM, Gregor P, Spviak C, Uhl GR. Mu-opiate receptor: cDNA cloning and expression. Proceedings of the National Academy of Sciences. 1993:90:10,230-10,234.

38. Chen Y, Mestek A, Liu J, Yu L. Molecular cloning of a rat kappa opioid receptor reveals sequence similarities to the mu and delta opioid receptors. Biochemical Journal. 1993:295:625-628.

39. Meunier JC, Mollereau C, Toll L et al. Isolation and structure of the endogenous agonist of opioid receptor-like ORL$_1$ receptor. Nature. 1995:377:532-535.

40. Reinscheid RK, Nothacker HP, Bourson A et al. Orphanin FQ: a neuropeptide that activates an opioidlike G protein-coupled receptor. Science. 1995:270: 792-794.

41. Spangler R, Ho A, Zhou Y et al. Regulation of kappa opioid receptor mRNA in the rat brain by "binge" pattern cocaine administration and correlation with preprodynorphin mRNA. Mol Brain Res. 1996:38:71-76.

42. Branch AD, Unterwald EM, Lee SE, Kreek MJ. Quantitation of preproenkephalin mRNA levels in brain regions from male Fischer rats following chronic cocaine treatment using a recently developed solution hybridization procedure. Mol Brain Res. 1992: 14:231-238.

43. Unterwald EM, Rubenfeld JM, Imai Y et al. Chronic opioid antagonist administration upregulates mu opioid receptor binding without altering mu opioid receptor mRNA levels. Mol Brain Res. 1995:33:351-355.

44. Spangler R, Zhou Y, Unterwald EM, Kreek MJ. Opioid peptide and receptor mRNA levels in the rat brain determined by TCA precipitation of mRNA: cRNA hybrids. In: Harris LS, ed. Problems of Drug Dependence, 1994; Proceedings of the 56th Annual Scientific Meeting of the College on Problems of Drug Dependence. Rockville, MD: NIDA Research Monograph Series, NIH Publication No. 95-3883. 1995:153:484.

45. Spangler R, Unterwald EM, Branch A et al. Chronic cocaine administration increases prodynorphin mRNA levels in the caudate putamen of rats. In: Harris LS, ed. Problems of Drug Dependence, 1992; Proceedings of the 54th Annual Scientific Meeting of the College on Problems of Drug Dependence Rockville, MD: NIDA Research Monograph Series, DHHS Publication No. (ADM) 93-3505. 1993:132:142.

46. Spangler R, Unterwald EM, Kreek MJ. 'Binge' cocaine administration induces a sustained increase of prodynorphin mRNA in rat caudate-putamen. Mol Brain Res. 1993: 19:323-327.

47. Zhou Y, Spangler R, Ho A et al. Corticotropin-releasing hormone (CRH) mRNA diurnal rhythms in rat hypothalamus and frontal cortex and inhibition by dexamethasone. In: Harris LS, ed. Problems of Drug Dependence, 1994; Proceedings of the 56th Annual Scientific Meeting of the College on Problems of Drug Dependence. Rockville, MD: NIDA Research Monograph Series, NIH Publication No. 95-3883. 1995:153:114.

48. Zhou Y, Spangler R, LaForge KS, Kreek MJ. Attenuation of the hypothalamic-pituitary-adrenal response to chronic "binge" pattern cocaine administration corresponds to decreased CRH mRNA in rat hypothalamus. Regulatory Peptides: Proceedings of the 25th International Narcotics Research Conference. 1994:54:345-346.

49. Zhou Y, Spangler R, LaForge KS et al. Regulation of POMC gene expression in rat pituitary, hypothalamus and amygdala by chronic administration of CRH, dex, and methadone. In: Harris LS, ed. Problems of Drug Dependence, 1995; Proceedings of the 57th Annual Scientific Meeting of the College on Problems of Drug Dependence. Rockville, MD: NIDA Research Monograph Series. Publication No. 96-4116. 1996:162:183.

50. Zhou Y, Spangler R, LaForge KS et al. Modulation of CRF-R1 mRNA in rat anterior pituitary by dexamethasone: correlation with POMC mRNA. Peptides. 1996:17:435-441.

51. Kreek MJ. Effects of opiates, opioid antagonists, and cocaine on the endogenous opioid system: clinical and laboratory studies. In: Harris LS, ed. Problems of Drug Dependence, 1991: Proceedings of the 53rd Annual Scientific Meeting, The Committee on Problems of Drug Dependence, Inc. Rockville, MD: NIDA Monograph, DHHS Publication No.(ADM) 92-1888. 1992:119:44-48.

52. Moldow RL, Fischman AJ. Cocaine induced secretion of ACTH, beta-endorphin and corticosterone. Peptides. 1987:8:819-822.

53. Sarnyai Z, Biro E, Penke B, Telegdy G. The cocaine-induced elevation of plasma corticosterone is mediated by endogenous corticotropin-releasing factor (CRF) in rats. Brain Res. 1992:589:154-156.

54. Mello NK, Sarnyai Z, Mendelson JH et al. Acute effects of cocaine on anterior pituitary hormones in male and female rhesus monkeys. Journal of Pharmacological Experimental Therapy. 1993:266:804-811.

55. Rivier C, Lee S. Stimulatory effect of cocaine on ACTH secretion: role of the hypothalamus. Mol. and Cell. Neurosciences. 1994:5:189-195.

56. Mello NK, Sarnyai Z, Mendelson JH et al. Acute effects of cocaine on anterior pituitary hormones in ovariectomized female rhesus monkeys. Journal of Pharmacological Experimental Therapy. 1995:272:1059-1066.

57. Kreek MJ. Medical complications in methadone patients. Ann NY Acad Sci. 1978:311:110-134.

58. Kreek MJ, Wardlaw SL, Friedman J et al. Effects of chronic exogenous opioid administration on levels of one endogenous opioid (beta-endorphin) in man. In: Simon E and Takagi H, eds. Advances in Endogenous and Exogenous Opioids. Tokyo, Japan: Kodansha Ltd. Publishers. 1981:364-366.

59. Kreek MJ, Hartman N. Chronic use of opioids and antipsychotic drugs: Side effects, effects on endogenous opioids and toxicity. Ann NY Acad Sci. 1982:398:151-172.

60. Kreek MJ, Wardlaw SL, Hartman N et al. Circadian rhythms and levels of beta-endorphin, ACTH, and cortisol during chronic methadone maintenance treatment in humans. Life Sciences, Sup. I. 1983:33:409-411.

61. Kreek MJ, Raghunath J, Plevy S et al. ACTH, cortisol and beta-endorphin response to metyrapone testing during chronic methadone maintenance treatment in humans. Neuropeptides. 1984:5:277-278.

62. Kosten TR, Kreek MJ, Swift C et al. Beta-endorphin levels in CSF during methadone maintenance. Life Sciences. 1987:41:1071-1076.

63. Kennedy JA, Hartman N, Sbriglio R et al. Metyrapone-induced withdrawal symptoms. Brit J Addict. 1990: 85:1133-1140.

64. Kosten TR, Morgan C, Kreek MJ. Beta-endorphin levels during heroin, methadone, buprenorphine and naloxone challenges: Preliminary findings. Biolog Psych. 1992:32:523-528.

65. Kreek MJ. Tolerance and dependence: Implications for the pharmacological treatment of addiction. In: Harris LS, ed. Problems of Drug Dependence, 1986; Proceedings of the 48th Annual Scientific Meeting of The Committee on Problems of Drug Dependence. Rockville, MD: NIDA Research Monograph Series, DHHS Publication No.(ADM) 87-1508. 1987:76:53-61.

66. Cushman P, Kreek MJ. Some endocrinologic observations in narcotic addicts. In: Zimmerman E and George R, eds. Narcotic and the Hypothalamus. New York: Raven Press. 1974:161-173.

67. Tabasco-Minguillan J, Novick DM, Kreek MJ. Liver function tests in nonparenteral cocaine users. In: Harris LS, ed. Problems of Drug Dependence, 1990; Proceedings of the 52nd Annual Scientific Meeting of the Committee on Problems of Drug Dependence. Rockville, MD: NIDA Research Monograph Series, DHHS Publication No. (ADM) 91-1753. 1991:105:372.

68. Kreek MJ. Multiple drug abuse patterns: Recent trends and associated medical consequences. Advances in Substance Abuse: Behavioral and Biological Research. London, England: Jessica Kingsley Publishers Ltd. 1991:4:91-111.

69. Unterwald EM, Horne-King J, Kreek MJ. Chronic cocaine alters brain mu opioid receptors. Brain Res. 1992:584:314-318.

70. Unterwald EM, Cox BM, Kreek MJ et al. Chronic repeated cocaine administration alters basal and opioid-regulated adenylyl cyclase activity. Synapse. 1993:15:33-38.

71. Maisonneuve IM, Kreek MJ. Acute tolerance to the dopamine response induced by a binge pattern of cocaine administration in male rats: An *in vivo* microdialysis study. J Pharmacol and Exp Therapeutics. 1994:268(2):916-921.

72. Unterwald EM, Rubenfeld JM, Kreek MJ. Repeated cocaine administration upregulates k and μ, but not δ, opioid receptors. NeuroReport. 1994: 5:1613-1616.

73. Unterwald EM, Ho A, Rubenfeld JM, Kreek MJ. Time course of the development of behavioral sensitization and dopamine receptor upregulation during binge cocaine administration. J Pharmacol and Exp Therapeutics. 1994:270(3): 1387-1397.

74. Maisonneuve IM, Ho A, Kreek MJ. Chronic administration of a cocaine "binge" alters basal extracellular levels in male rats: An *in vivo* microdialysis study. J Pharmacol and Exp Therapeutics. 1995:272:652-657.

75. Maggos CE, Spangler R, Zhou Y, Kreek MJ. Dopamine transporter mRNA levels in the rat substantia nigra and ventral tegmental area immediately following and at two days and ten days after 'binge' cocaine administration. In: Harris LS, ed. Problems of Drug Dependence, 1994; Proceedings of the 56th Annual Scientific Meeting of the College on Problems of Drug Dependence. Rockville, MD: NIDA Research Monograph Series, NIH Publication No. 95-3883. 1995:153:508.

76. Maggos CE, Spangler R, Zhou Y et al. Quantification of dopamine transporter mRNA in rat brain and modulations by dopamine receptor antagonists and cocaine. In: Harris LS, ed. NIDA Research Monograph Series, Problems of Drug Dependence, 1995; Proceedings of the 57th Annual Scientific Meeting of the College on Problems of Drug Dependence. Publication No. 96-4116. 1996:162:218.

77. Claye LH, Unterwald EM, Ho A, Kreek MJ. Both dynorphin A_{1-17} and [des-tyr^1] dynorphin A_{2-17} inhibit adenylyl cyclase activity in rat caudate putamen. J Pharmacol and Exp Therapeutics. 1996 (in press).

78. Kreek MJ, Ho A, Borg L. Dynorphin A_{1-13} administration causes elevation of serum levels of prolactin in human subjects. In: Harris LS, ed. Problems of Drug Dependence, 1993; proceedings of the 55th Annual Scientific Meeting of the College on Problems of Drug dependence. Rockville, MD: NIDA Research Monograph Series, NIH Publication No. 94-3749.1 141:108, 1994.

79. Chou JZ, Pinto S, Kreek MJ, Chait BT. Study of opioid peptides by laser desorption mass spectrometry. In: Harris LS, ed. Problems of Drug Dependence, 1992; Proceedings of the 54th Annual Scientific Meeting of the College on Problems of Drug Dependence. Rockville, MD: NIDA Research Monograph Series, DHHS Publication No. (ADM) 93-3505. 1993:132:380.

80. Chou JZ, Maisonneuve IM, Chait BT, Kreek MJ. Study of dynorphin A(1-17) *in vivo* processing in rat brain by microdialysis and matrix-assisted laser desorption mass spectrometry. In: Harris LS, ed. Problems of Drug Dependence, 1993; Proceedings of the 55th Annual Scientific Meeting of the College on Problems of Drug Dependence. Rockville, MD: NIDA Research Monograph Series, NIH Publication No. 94-3749. 1994:141:240.

81. Chou JZ, Kreek MJ, Chait BT. Matrix-assisted laser desorption mass spectrometry of biotransformation products of dynorphin A *in vitro*. J Am Soc Mass Spectrom. 1994:5:10-16.

82. Chou JZ, Chait BT, Kreek MJ. Study of dynorphin A peptides *in vitro* processing in human blood by matrix-assisted laser desorption mass spectrometry. In: Harris LS, ed. Problems of Drug Dependence, 1994; Proceedings of the 56th Annual Scientific Meeting of the College on Problems of Drug Dependence. Rockville, MD: NIDA Research Monograph Series, NIH Publication No. 95-3883. 1995:153:252.

83. Butelman ER, Yu J, Chou JZ et al. Dynorphin A (1-13): Biotransformation in human and rhesus monkey blood and antinociception. In: Harris LS, ed. Problems of Drug Dependence, 1995; Proceedings of the 57th Annual Scientific Meet-

ing of the College on Problems of Drug Dependence. NIH Publication No. 96-4116. 1996:162:225.

84. Yu J, Butelman ER, Woods JH et al. Studies of *in vitro* processing of dynorphin A (1-17) in human blood and in rhesus monkey blood. In: Harris LS, ed. Problems of Drug Dependence, 1995; Proceedings of the 57th Annual Scientific Meeting of the College on Problems of Drug Dependence. NIH Publication No. 96-4116. 1996:162:131.

Pattern of Cocaine Use
in Methadone-Maintained Individuals
Applying for Research Studies

Frances Rudnick Levin, MD
Richard W. Foltin, PhD
Marian W. Fischman, PhD

SUMMARY. Twenty-three methadone-maintained individuals seeking admission into a cocaine study were interviewed using the Pattern-of-Drug-Use assessment. Sample characteristics included: 96% male, 91% Caucasian, and 36 ± 5 mean years of age. Mean methadone dose was 81 ± 20 mg. On average, subjects reported using greater than $200 or 5 grams of cocaine per week. "Binge/crash" cocaine use did not appear to be the typical pattern of use. However, during daily periods of cocaine use, repeated injections of large amounts of cocaine were taken, which may place patients at risk for medical complications. These findings emphasize the importance of developing novel treatment strategies to treat these dually-addicted

Frances Rudnick Levin, Richard W. Foltin, and Marian W. Fischman are affiliated with the Division on Substance Abuse, New York State Psychiatric Institute and Department of Psychiatry, College of Physicians and Surgeons of Columbia University, New York, NY.

Address correspondence to: Frances Rudnick Levin, MD, Division on Substance Abuse, New York State Psychiatric Institute and Department of Psychiatry, College of Physicians and Surgeons of Columbia University, 722 West 168th Street, Unit 66, New York, NY 10032.

[Haworth co-indexing entry note]: "Pattern of Cocaine Use in Methadone-Maintained Individuals Applying for Research Studies." Levin, Frances Rudnick, Richard W. Foltin, and Marian W. Fischman. Co-published simultaneously in *Journal of Addictive Diseases* (The Haworth Medical Press, an imprint of The Haworth Press, Inc.) Vol. 15, No. 4, 1996, pp. 97-106; and: *The Neurobiology of Cocaine Addiction: From Bench to Bedside* (ed: Herman Joseph, and Barry Stimmel) The Haworth Medical Press, an imprint of The Haworth Press, Inc., 1996, pp. 97-106. Single or multiple copies of this article are available for a fee from The Haworth Document Delivery Service [1-800-342-9678, 9:00 a.m. - 5:00 p.m. (EST). E-mail address: getinfo@haworth.com].

individuals. *[Article copies available for a fee from The Haworth Document Delivery Service: 1-800-342-9678. E-mail address: getinfo@haworth. com]*

INTRODUCTION

Although cocaine use by patients maintained on methadone is not new,[1,2] the rapid rise of cocaine use among this population has greatly concerned clinicians working within methadone treatment settings.[3] In a survey of 24 methadone programs, the percentage of methadone-maintained patients who used cocaine ranged from 0-40%.[4] The finding that some patients initiate cocaine use only after entering methadone treatment[5,6] is unquestionably worrisome. Additionally, cocaine use by methadone patients has been associated with increased criminality,[7] treatment failure,[8] and risk for HIV infection.[9]

Possible reasons for combined methadone and cocaine use include: (1) the minimization of side effects from one drug by the use of the other (e.g., methadone reduces the jitteriness associated with cocaine use), (2) enhanced or novel subjective effect produced by combined use, and (3) the lack of specific interactions between opiates and cocaine; instead, the increased availability and purity of cocaine has led to an escalation of use among methadone-maintained patients. Depending on the patient and region of the country, one or more of these reasons might apply. Simply documenting the presence or absence of cocaine use in methadone patients is not sufficient when attempting to assess the magnitude of the problem. More in-depth evaluation methods deserve further exploration. As reviewed by Kidorf and Stitzer,[10] assessment techniques have included frequency prevalence data, drug use severity scores based on frequency data, DSM-IV criteria for cocaine abuse and/or dependence, or urinalysis testing. These investigators found that methadone-maintained patients in their clinic population generally use relatively low amounts of cocaine (approximately 0.8 g/week) compared to non-opioid dependent patients applying for cocaine treatment programs. Surprisingly, with the exception of the study by Kidorf and Stitzer,[10] there is little detailed information regarding the pattern of cocaine use among methadone-maintained patients.

Subjects applying for our research study reported that 1 gram of cocaine costs $35-$60. Thus, individuals receiving methadone within the NYC area may continue to abuse cocaine even when they are pharmacologically treated for their opiate addiction, in part, because cocaine is both cheap and widely available. It was our impression that the methadone-maintained subjects applying for our residential cocaine study in NYC had a different pattern of cocaine use than the pattern described by Kidorf and Stitzer[10] in their Baltimore sample of patients. The purpose of this study was to determine the monthly, weekly, and daily pattern of cocaine and other drug use in this self-selected population.

METHODS

Subjects and Intake Process

Twenty-three consecutively self-referred cocaine-using methadone-maintained subjects applying for participation between July 1993 and June 1994 for an inpatient research protocol evaluating the behavioral and physiological effects of cocaine were assessed with the Pattern-of-Drug-Use assessment. Subjects were recruited by newspaper and radio advertisements. In addition, one of the senior investigators and research nurses visited several methadone programs and described the protocol to assembled groups of methadone staff members. All subjects were prescreened by telephone. Potential subjects were repeatedly evaluated by several staff members, including the research psychiatrist (FRL), to determine whether they were interested in treatment for their cocaine addiction. If they expressed interest in cocaine abuse treatment, a referral was made, and they were not accepted into the study.

The intake process generally occurred over several days. The inclusion criteria for the research protocol were: (1) current maintenance on methadone, and (2) use of intravenous cocaine within the past 30 days. Exclusion criteria were: (1) current physiologic dependence on any psychoactive substance(s) other than methadone, opiates, cocaine, or nicotine, (2) medical or psychiatric problems that made individuals ineligible for the research protocol, or (3) current legal problems. Results from medical tests which would exclude subjects from the research protocol were usually not determined prior to carrying out the Pattern-of-Drug-Use assessment. In addition, the Pattern-of-Drug-Use assessment was carried out conjointly with the physical and psychiatric evaluation. Thus, subjects with physical problems were not necessarily excluded.

Data Collection and Analysis

All subjects were interviewed by the research psychiatrist, or one of the research psychiatric fellows, regarding their substance use over the previous 28 days. Similar to an earlier study,[11] part of this interview involved presenting the subject with a sheet of paper divided into a seven column by five row square grid representing a blank calendar. The current day of the week and the past 28 days on the calendar were identified. Subjects then indicated significant events during the past 28 days that might be useful in providing reference points (e.g., paydays, holidays, birthdays). Then, beginning with the day before the interview and working backwards, subjects were asked to indicate on which days drugs were taken. First, subjects were asked to recall daily methadone intake, since patterns of methadone use were generally more stable than other drugs used, and missed days were remembered more easily. This procedure was repeated for cocaine, and then for any other drug used in the past 28 days.

An additional component of the Pattern-of-Drug-Use assessment consisted of the subject describing his/her typical pattern of drug use during a 24-hour period. A grid consisting of 24 rows (one for each hour) and 9 columns listing various classes of abusable substances was shown to each subject. Working with the subject, the research psychiatrist ascertained the subject's typical daily use pattern. If the weekend use was different than daily use, this was documented.

RESULTS

Sample Characteristics

The sample consisted of 23 methadone-maintained individuals: mean age of 36 ± 5 years, 91% Caucasian, 96% male. Because recruitment was often by "word-of-mouth," this might have led to an increased homogeneity of the sample. None of the subjects were married, and less than 20% were currently employed. Average methadone dose was 81 ± 20 mg. Fewer than 25% of the subjects spent greater than 2 months of their lifetime in jail, with an average of 49 ± 125 days. The subjects had a mean education of 13 ± 1 years. All of the subjects were "research naive." The average age of onset of heroin use was slightly younger than cocaine use (20 versus 22 years). Interestingly, 2 subjects reported a period of heavy regular cocaine use (i.e., at least once a week) prior to the age of their first heroin use.

Monthly Frequency of Cocaine and Other Drug Use

Figure 1 compares the average number of days of use of various psychoactive substances over the 28 days prior to initial interview. Less than one-third of the subjects missed any of their methadone doses, with days

FIGURE 1. Mean days of use (± SD) for various psychoactive drugs in the 28 days prior to evaluation for 23 methadone-maintained cocaine abusers applying for a research cocaine study.

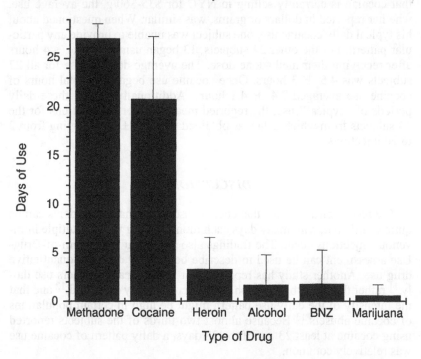

of receiving methadone averaging 27 ± 1.5. Most subjects reported almost daily cocaine use (mean 21 ± 6 days). Despite receiving adequate doses of methadone, almost 75% admitted to using heroin in the past month; however, for the entire sample, average days of use were 3 ± 3 days, with only 2 subjects using heroin ≥ 10 days. Similarly, psychoactive substance use, other than cocaine, was low with average days of use totaling less than 2 for any other substance. Frequent concurrent drug use, defined as the specific use of another drug or drug combination during at least 50% of the days that cocaine was also used, was uncommon; only 2 out of the 12 subjects who used benzodiazepines reported frequent concurrent use.

Weekly and Daily Pattern of Cocaine Use

Subjects were also asked to quantitate their weekly amount of cocaine use. Some individuals felt that they could be more "accurate" if they described their weekly use in dollars, whereas others preferred to report their use in grams. For 2 subjects, quantitative data were not available. Average amount of cocaine use was $255 ± $144 or 5.3 ± 3.0 g. Given that cocaine is currently selling in NYC for $35-$60/g, the average use, whether reported in dollars or grams, was similar. When questioned about his typical daily cocaine use, one subject was unable to provide any particular pattern. For the other 22 subjects, 13 began using cocaine ≤4 hours after receiving their methadone dose. The average delay in use for all 22 subjects was 4.5 ± 3 hours. Once cocaine use began, the total hours of cocaine use averaged 7.4 ± 4.1 hours. Additionally, during these daily periods of "typical" use, the reported mean number of injections for the 14 subjects from which data was obtained was 6.9 ± 4.8, ranging from 2 to 20 injections.

DISCUSSION

The results clearly show that cocaine use by methadone patients can be quite significant, with many days each month during which multiple intravenous injections occur. The findings also show that the Pattern-of-Drug-Use assessment can be used to describe both qualitative and quantitative drug use. Another study has reported that some cocaine abusers use daily,[11] rather than the "binge/crash" pattern previously described,[12] and that the intensity of the daily use pattern might be high in certain populations of cocaine abusers.[13] Because almost two-thirds of the subjects reported using cocaine at least 23 out of the 28 days, a daily pattern of cocaine use was relatively common.

In addition to examining monthly and weekly patterns of cocaine use, we were interested in our subjects' daily pattern of use. Interestingly, most use cocaine within 4-5 hours of receiving their methadone dose, and use, on average, at least 7 hours a day. Thus, most start using cocaine early in the afternoon, spending most of their day taking large quantities of cocaine. Although none of the patients entering our residential research study were on doses greater than 100 mg of methadone, most of our applicants were receiving doses of methadone well above the minimum amount found to be effective in reducing heroin use.[4] Thus, it does not appear that adequate, or relatively high, doses of methadone "block" cocaine use.

However, similar to Arndt et al.'s study,[14] our subjects reported little additional opiate use. Most subjects used heroin at least once during the past 4 weeks, but average use was less than 4 days. This is not surprising given the sample's average methadone dose (81 mg). Besides cocaine use, there was not a substantial amount of other drug use among these methadone-maintained patients. Only 2 subjects reported using another class of substances (i.e., benzodiazepines) along with cocaine on a regular basis. Although almost half of the subjects reported using alcohol in the past 28 days, none routinely used alcohol with cocaine. This probably does not represent a "typical" alcohol use pattern for cocaine-abusing methadone-maintained patients. Because physiologic dependence on alcohol and sedatives/hypnotics was an exclusion criteria for admission, one might expect to see greater alcohol and other drug use in cocaine-abusing methadone-maintained patients being evaluated in clinical settings. However, for this sample, it does not appear that alcohol is being used to modulate the effects of cocaine. Thus, it is unlikely that reducing alcohol use, perhaps by administering antabuse, would make a significant impact on cocaine use in this population.

Compared to Kidorf and Stitzer,[10] who reported that their methadone-maintained patients take cocaine an average of 3 days per week, our subjects reported an average of 22 days in the past 4 weeks. The difference in extent of use might be accounted for by the different methodologies employed. Whereas Kidorf and Stitzer[10] obtained data for a single one-week period, we obtained data for the past month. We required subjects to report in a detailed fashion their drug use for the past 28 days, but did not repeat the interview and obtain urine test results as Kidorf and Stitzer[10] had done since our data was collected retrospectively. This is clearly a limitation of this study. Other limitations include the small sample size and the nature of our sample. The subjects consisted primarily of Caucasian males; women and minority populations in methadone programs might have distinctly different patterns of cocaine and other drug use. However, recently, Ziedonis et al.[15] found that among cocaine abusers seeking treatment, African-American patients did not show a different frequency of use than Caucasian patients.

Another reason to explain the "discrepancy" between our findings and that of Kidorf and Stitzer's[10] may be the variance in cost and availability of cocaine in different US cities. Kidorf and Stitzer[10] estimated that based on 0.1 g = $10 or a "dime bag," their Baltimore patients used, on average, 0.82 g/week of cocaine. This cost/gram is substantially greater than what is reported by our patients; the lower cost of cocaine in NYC might facilitate heavier use among the methadone-maintained subjects evaluated in our study. A further explanation for the greater frequency of use in our study might be due to the detailed method of obtaining monthly patterns of use. Subjects might "overstate" their frequency of use in order to ensure entry into our study.

It is worrisome that there is a subpopulation of methadone-maintained patients who are repeatedly injecting themselves with large amounts of cocaine on a daily basis. Cocaine use may be sabotaging one of the major goals of methadone treatment, that is, allowing patients to lead productive lives. Therefore, recognition of the extent of cocaine use in methadone programs is the first step. The next is to develop effective strategies to combat dual-addiction. Strategies which have been used to treat cocaine abusers include: (1) positive contingency contracting,[16] (2) relapse prevention,[17] and (3) a wide range of pharmacotherapies.[18] However, no one approach has been shown to have clear-cut efficacy with cocaine abusers. Instead, combined approaches which are individualized for different subpopulations need to be developed. For cocaine-abusing methadone-maintained patients, these approaches have been applied with limited success.[14,19] Some investigators have found that buprenorphine, a partial opiate agonist, may be useful for this dually-addicted population;[20,21] however, more recent controlled studies with dually-dependent patients have failed to show a significant reduction in cocaine use.[22] McLellan et al.[23] found that methadone-maintained patients who received minimal treatment services were less likely to have extended periods of cocaine abstinence compared to those receiving standard or enhanced services. Thus, the trend in methadone programs needs to be towards an enhancement, rather than a reduction in treatment services if cocaine use is to be reduced.

As this study demonstrates, similar to other findings, cocaine is heavily used by a subgroup of patients in methadone-maintenance programs. These patients no longer have a "primary" opiate addiction. Instead, their amount of cocaine use and time spent using cocaine impedes their ability to work productively, and increases their risk of physical complications associated with intravenous cocaine use. Clearly, methadone programs need to develop strategies to combat this problem, since it is subverting the effectiveness of methadone treatment.

REFERENCES

1. Chambers CD, Taylor WJR, Moffett AD. The incidence of cocaine abuse among methadone maintenance patients. Int J Addict. 1972; 7:427-441.

2. Strug DL, Hunt DE, Goldsmith DS, Lipton DS, Spunt B. Patterns of cocaine use among methadone clients. Int J Addict. 1985; 20:1163-1175.

3. Cushman P. Cocaine use in a population of drug abusers on methadone. Hosp Commun Psychiatry. 1988; 39:1205-1207.

4. U.S. General Accounting Office. Methadone maintenance: some treatment programs are not effective. Greater federal oversight needed. Washington, D.C.:Government Printing Office, 1990; Publication no. GAO/HRD-90-104.

5. Hanbury R, Sturiano V, Cohen M, Stimmel B, Aguillaume C. Cocaine use in persons on methadone maintenance. Advances in Alcohol Substance Abuse. 1986; 6:197-206.

6. Chaisson RE, Bacchetti P, Osmond D, Brodie B, Sande MA, Moss AR. Cocaine use and HIV infection intravenous drug users in San Francisco. J Am Med Assoc. 1989; 261:561-565.

7. Hunt DE, Strug DL, Goldsmith DS, Lipton DS, Spunt B, Truitt L, Robertson, KA. An instant shot of "aah": cocaine use among methadone clients. J Psychoact Drugs. 1984; 16:217-227.

8. Black JL, Dolan MP, Penk WE, Robinowitz WE, DeFord HA. The effects of increased cocaine use on drug treatment. Addict Behav. 1987; 12:289-292.

9. Hartgers C, Van Den Hoek A, Krijnen P, Van Brussel GHA, Coutinho RA. Changes over time in heroin and cocaine use among injecting drug users in Amsterdam, the Netherlands, 1985-1989. Br J Addiction. 1991; 86:1091-1097.

10. Kidorf M and Stitzer ML. Descriptive analysis of cocaine use of methadone patients. Drug Alcohol Depend. 1993; 32:267-275.

11. Levin FR, Hess JM, Gorelick DA, Kreiter NA, Fudala PJ. Patterns of cocaine use among cocaine-dependent outpatients. Am J Addictions. 1993; 2: 109-115.

12. Gawin FH and Kleber HD. Abstinence symptomatology and psychiatric diagnosis in cocaine abusers. Arch Gen Psychiatry. 1986; 43:107-113.

13. Carroll KM and Rounsaville BJ. History and significance of childhood attention deficit disorder in treatment-seeking cocaine abusers. Compr Psychiatry. 1993; 34:75-86.

14. Arndt IO, Dorozynsky L, Woody GE, McLellan AT, O'Brien CP. Desipramine treatment of cocaine dependence in methadone-maintained patients. Arch Gen Psychiatry. 1992; 49:888-893.

15. Ziedonis DM, Rayford BS, Bryant KJ, Rounsaville BJ. Psychiatric comorbidity in white and African-American cocaine addicts seeking substance abuse treatment. Hosp Commun Psychiatry. 1994; 45:43-49.

16. Higgins ST, Budney AJ, Bickel WK, Hughes JR, Foerg F, Badger G. Achieving cocaine abstinence with a behavioral approach. Am J Psychiatry. 1993; 150:763-769.

17. Carroll KM, Rounsaville BJ, Gordon LT, Nich C, Jatlow P, Bisighini RM, Gawin, FH. Psychotherapy and pharmacotherapy for ambulatory cocaine abusers. Arch Gen Psychiatry. 1994; 51:177-187.

18. Kosten TR. Pharmacotherapies. In: Kosten TR and Kleber HD, eds. Clinician's guide to cocaine addiction: theory, research, and treatment. New York:The Guilford Press, 1992:273-289.

19. Magura S, Casriel C, Goldsmith DS, Strug DL, Lipton DS. Contingency contracting with polydrug-abusing methadone patients. Addict Behav. 1988; 13:113-118.

20. Mello NK, Mendelson JH, Lukas SE, Gastfriend DR, Teoh SK, Holman L. Buprenorphine treatment of opiate and cocaine abuse; clinical and preclinical studies. Harv Rev Psychiatry. 1993; 1:168-183.

21. Keystone TR, Morgan C, Kleber HD. Treatment of heroin addicts using buprenorphine. Am J Drug Alcohol Abuse. 1991; 17:119-128.

22. Strain EC, Preston KL, Stitzer ML, Liebson IA, Bigelow GE. The effects of cocaine in buprenorphine-maintained outpatient volunteers: results from clinical experience and laboratory challenges. Am J Addictions. 1994; 3:129-143.

23. McLellan AT, Arndt IO, Metzger DS, Woody GE, O'Brien CP. The effects of psychosocial services in substance abuse treatment. J Am Med Assoc. 1993; 269:1953-1959.

SELECTIVE GUIDE TO CURRENT REFERENCE SOURCES ON TOPICS DISCUSSED IN THIS ISSUE

Lynn Kasner Morgan, MLS

Each issue of *Journal of Addictive Diseases* features a section offering suggestions on where to look for further information on included topics. The intent is to guide readers to selective substantive sources of current information.

Some published reference works utilize designated terminology (controlled vocabularies) which must be used to find material on topics of interest. For these, a sample of available search terms has been indicated to assist the reader in accessing appropriate sources for his/her purposes. Other reference tools use keywords or free text terms from the title of the document, the abstract, and the name of any responsible agency or conference. In searching using keywords, be sure to look under all possible synonyms to retrieve the concept in question.

Lynn Kasner Morgan is Assistant Professor of Medical Education, Assistant Dean for Information Resources and Systems, and Director of the Gustave L. and Janet W. Levy Library of the Mount Sinai Medical Center, Inc., One Gustave L. Levy Place, New York, NY 10029-6574.

[Haworth co-indexing entry note]: "Selective Guide to Current Reference Sources on Topics Discussed in This Issue." Morgan, Lynn Kasner. Co-published simultaneously in *Journal of Addictive Diseases* (The Haworth Medical Press, an imprint of The Haworth Press, Inc.) Vol. 15, No. 4, 1996, pp. 107-118; and: *The Neurobiology of Cocaine Addiction: From Bench to Bedside* (ed: Herman Joseph, and Barry Stimmel) The Haworth Medical Press, an imprint of The Haworth Press, Inc., 1996, pp. 107-118. Single or multiple copies of this article are available for a fee from The Haworth Document Delivery Service [1-800-342-9678, 9:00 a.m. - 5:00 p.m. (EST). E-mail address: getinfo@ haworth.com].

An asterisk (*) appearing before a published source indicates that all or part of that source is in machine-readable form and can be accessed through an online database search. Database searching is recommended for retrieving sources of information that coordinate multiple variables, concepts, or subject areas. Most health sciences libraries offer database services which can include mediated online searching, access to locally mounted datafiles, front-end software packages, and CD-ROM technology. Searching can also be done from one's office or home with subscriptions to database service vendors and microcomputers equipped with modems.

Interactive electronic communications systems, such as electronic mail, discussion groups, bulletin boards, and receiving and transferring files are available through the Internet, which offers timely and global information resources in all disciplines, including the health sciences. Some groups which might be of interest are: ALCOHOL (ALCOHOL@LMUACAD), DRUG ABUSE (DRUGABUS@UMAB), 12STEP@TRWRB.DSD.COM and ADDICTION MEDICINE (MAJORDOMO@AVOCADO.PC.HELSINKI. FI). The National Clearinghouse for Alcohol and Drug Information Center for Substance Abuse Prevention maintains PREVline, a bulletin board for alcohol and drug information. There are also many sites with World Wide Web pages which can be reached by individuals with a Web browser such as Mosaic or Netscape. A suggested starting point is http://www.yahoo.com/health, Web Crawler searching tool http://webcrawler.com or World Wide Web Worm http://wwwmcb.cs.colorado.edu/home/mcbryan/www.html.

Readers are encouraged to consult their librarians for further assistance before undertaking research on a topic.

Suggestions regarding the content and organization of this section are welcome and should be sent to the author.

1. INDEXING AND ABSTRACTING SOURCES

Place of publication, publisher, start date, frequency of publication, and brief descriptions are noted.

Biological Abstracts (1926-) and *Biological Abstracts/RRM* (v.18, 1980-). Philadelphia, BioSciences Information Service, semimonthly. Reports on worldwide research in the life sciences.

> See: Concept headings for abstracts, such as behavioral biology, pharmacology, psychiatry, public health, and toxicology sections.

> See: Keyword-in-context subject index.

Chemical Abstracts. Columbus, Ohio, American Chemical Society, 1907- , weekly. A key to the world's literature of chemistry and chemical engineering, including serial publications, proceedings and edited collections, technical reports, dissertations, new book and audiovisual materials announcements, and patent documents.

See: *Index Guide* for cross-referencing and indexing policies.

See: *General Subject Index* terms, such as drug dependence, drug-drug interactions, drug tolerance.
See: Keyword subject indexes.

Dissertation Abstracts International. Section A. The Humanities and Social Sciences and *Section B. The Sciences and Engineering.* Ann Arbor, Mich., University Microfilms, v.30, 1969/70- , monthly. Includes author-prepared abstracts of doctoral dissertations from 500 participating institutions throughout North America and the world. A separate section contains European dissertations.

See: Keyword subject index.

Excerpta Medica. Amsterdam, The Netherlands, Excerpta Medica Foundation, 1947- , 42 subject sections.

A major abstracting service covering more than 4,300 biomedical journals. The abstracts, including English summaries for non-English-language articles, appear in one or more of the published subject sections, excluding Section 38, *Adverse Reactions Titles,* which is an index only. Each of the sections has a comprehensive subject index. Since 1978 all the *Excerpta Medica* sections have been available for computer searching in the integrated online file, EMBASE.

Particularly relevant to the topics in this issue are Section 40, *Drug Dependence, Alcohol Abuse and Alcoholism;* and the sections that have addiction, alcoholism, or drug subdivisions: Section 30, *Clinical and Experimental Pharmacology*; Section 32, *Psychiatry*; and Section 17, *Public Health, Social Medicine and Epidemiology.*

Hospital and Health Administration Index. Chicago, American Hospital Association, v. 51, 1995- , 3 times per year, with annual cumulations. Formerly the Hospital Literature Index, v.13, 1957- v.50, 1994. Published as the primary guide to literature on the organization and administration of hospitals and other health care providers, the financing and delivery of health care, the development and implementation of health policy and reform, and health planning and research.

See: *MeSH* terms, such as alcoholism, cocaine, informed consent, smoking, substance abuse treatment centers.

Index Medicus (includes *Bibliography of Medical Reviews*). Bethesda, Md., National Library of Medicine, 1960- , monthly, with annual cumulations. Published as author and subject indexes to more than 3,000 journals in the biomedical sciences. Subject headings are based on the controlled vocabulary or thesaurus, *Medical Subject Headings (MeSH)*. Since 1966 it has been produced from the MEDLARS database, which provides more comprehensive retrieval, including keyword access and English-language abstracts, than its printed counterparts: *Index Medicus, International Nursing Index,* and *Index to Dental Literature.*

See: *MeSH* terms, such as alcohol drinking; alcoholism; behavior, addictive; cocaine; informed consent; interview, psychological; methadone; smoking; substance abuse; substance dependence; substance withdrawal syndrome; urinalysis.

Index to Scientific Reviews. Philadelphia, Institute for Scientific Information, 1974- , semiannual.

See: Permuterm keyword subject index.

See: Citation index.

International Pharmaceutical Abstracts. Washington, D.C., American Society of Hospital Pharmacists, 1964- , semimonthly. A key to the world's literature of pharmacy.

See: IPA subject terms, such as alcoholism, controlled substances, dependence, drug abuse, drug withdrawal, methadone, opiates, smoking, sociology.

See: Subject sections: legislation, laws and regulations; sociology, economics and ethics; toxicology.

Psychological Abstracts. Washington, D.C., American Psychological Association, 1927- , monthly. A compilation of nonevaluative summaries of the world's literature in psychology and related disciplines.

See: Index terms, such as addiction, alcoholism, alcohol rehabilitation, cocaine, drug abuse, drug addiction, drug dependency, drug rehabilitation, drug usage, drug usage screening, heroin addiction, informed consent, interviewing, methadone, tobacco smoking, treatment outcomes, urinalysis.

Public Affairs Information Service Bulletin. New York, Public Affairs Information Service, v.55, 1969- , semimonthly. An index to library material in the field of public affairs and public policy published throughout the world.

See: PAIS subject headings, such as alcoholism, cocaine, drug abuse, drug addicts, drugs, heroin, informed consent, methadone, narcotics, opium, smoking.

Science Citation Index. Philadelphia, Institute for Scientific Information, 1961- , bimonthly.

See: Permuterm keyword subject index.

See: Citation index.

Social Planning/Policy & Development Abstracts. San Diego, Calif., Sociological Abstracts, Inc., v.6, 1984- , semiannual.

See: Thesaurus and descriptors listed under *Sociological Abstracts.*

Social Work Abstracts. New York, National Association of Social Workers, v.13, 1977- , quarterly.

See: Subject index.

Sociological Abstracts. San Diego, Calif., Sociological Abstracts, Inc., 1952- , 6 times per year. A collection of nonevaluative abstracts which reflect the world's serial literature in sociology and related disciplines.

See: *Thesaurus of Sociological Indexing Terms.*

See: Descriptors such as addict/addicts/addictive/addiction, alcohol abuse, alcoholism, cocaine, drinking behavior, drug abuse, drug addiction, drug use, heroin, informed consent, interviews, opiates, smoking, substance abuse, tobacco.

2. CURRENT AWARENESS PUBLICATIONS

Current Contents: Clinical Medicine. Philadelphia, Institute for Scientific Information, v.15, 1987- , weekly.

> See: Keyword index.

Current Contents: Life Sciences. Philadelphia, Institute for Scientific Information, v. 10, 1967-, weekly.

> See: Keyword index.

Current Contents: Social & Behavioral Sciences. Philadelphia, Institute for Scientific Information, v.6, 1974- , weekly.

> See: Keyword index.

3. BOOKS

Medical and Health Care Books and Serials in Print: An Index to Literature in the Health Sciences. New York, R. R. Bowker Co., annual.

> See: Library of Congress subject headings, such as alcoholism, cocaine, drug abuse, drugs, methadone, narcotic habit, rehabilitation, smoking, substance abuse, tobacco, urinalysis.

National Library of Medicine Current Catalog. Bethesda, Md., National Library of Medicine, 1966- , quarterly, with annual cumulations.

> See: MeSH terms as noted in Section 1 under *Index Medicus.*

O'Brien, Robert [and others]. The Encyclopedia of Drug Abuse. 2nd ed. New York, Facts on File, c1992.

Stimmel, Barry [and others]. *The Facts About Drug Use: Coping with Drug Use in Your Family, at Work, in Your Community.* Mount Vernon, N.Y., Consumers' Union, c1991.

Substance Abuse: The Nation's Number One Health Problem. Key Indicators for Policy. Princeton, N.J., Robert Wood Johnson Foundation, 1993.

World Health Organization Catalogue: New Books. Geneva, World Health Organization, semiannual (supplements *World Health Organization Publications* and includes periodicals).

4. U.S. GOVERNMENT PUBLICATIONS

Alcohol and Other Drug Thesaurus: A Guide to Concepts and Terminology in Substance Abuse and Addiction (AOD Thesaurus). Rockville, Md., National Institute on Alcohol Abuse and Alcoholism, 1993.

See: Title keyword index.

*Monthly Catalog of United States Government Publications. Washington, D.C., U.S. Government Printing Office, 1895- , monthly.

See: Keyword index.

5. ONLINE BIBLIOGRAPHIC DATABASES

Only those databases which have no print counterparts are included in this section. Print sources which have online database equivalents are noted throughout this guide by the asterisk (*) which appears before the title. If you do not have direct access to these databases, consult your librarian for assistance.

ALCOHOL AND ALCOHOL PROBLEMS SCIENCE DATABASE: ETOH (National Institute on Alcohol Abuse and Alcoholism, Rockville, Md.).

Use: Keywords.

ALCOHOL INFORMATION FOR CLINICIANS AND EDUCATORS (Project Cork Institute, Dartmouth Medical School, Hanover, N.H.).

Use: Keywords.

AMERICAN STATISTICS INDEX (ASI) (Congressional Information Services, Inc., Washington, D.C.).

Use: Keywords.

DRUG INFORMATION FULLTEXT (American Society of Hospital Pharmacists, Bethesda, Md.).

Use: Keywords.

DRUGINFO AND ALCOHOL USE AND ABUSE (Hazelden Foundation, Center City, Minn., and Drug Information Service Center, College of Pharmacy, University of Minnesota, Minneapolis, Minn.).

    Use: Keywords.

LEXIS (Mead Data Central, Inc., Dayton, Ohio).

    Use: Guide library.

MAGAZINE INDEX (Information Access Co., Foster City, Calif.).

    Use: Keywords.

MENTAL HEALTH ABSTRACTS (MHA) (IFI/Plenum Data Co., Wilmington, NC).

    Use: Keywords.

NATIONAL NEWSPAPER INDEX (Information Access Co., Foster City, Calif.).

    Use: Keywords.

NTIS (Bibliographic Data Base, U.S. National Technical Information Service, Springfield, Va.).

    Use: Keywords.

PSYCINFO (American Psychological Association, Washington, D.C.).

    Use: Keywords.

WESTLAW (West Publishing Co., St. Paul, Minn.).

    Use: Keywords.

6. HANDBOOKS, DIRECTORIES, GRANT SOURCES, ETC.

Annual Register of Grant Support. Wilmette, Ill., National Register Pub. Co., annual.

See: Internal medicine; medicine; pharmacology, psychiatry, psychology, mental health sections.

See: Subject index.

Biomedical Index to PHS-Supported Research. Bethesda, Md., National Institutes of Health, Division of Research Grants, annual.

See: Subject index.

Database Directory. White Plains, N.Y., Knowledge Industry Publications in cooperation with the American Society for Information Science, annual.

See: Subject index.

Directory of Research Grants. Phoenix, Ariz., Oryx Press, annual.

See: Subject index terms, such as alcohol/alcoholism, cocaine, drugs/drug abuse, smoking behavior.

Encyclopedia of Associations. Detroit, Gale Research Co., annual (occasional supplements between editions).

See: Subject index.

Foundation Directory. New York, The Foundation Center, biennial (updated between editions by *Foundation Directory Supplement*).

See: Index of foundations.

See: Index of foundations by state and city.

See: Index of donors, trustees, and administrators.

See: Index of fields of interest.

Health Hotlines: Toll-Free Numbers from DIRLINE. Bethesda, Md., National Library of Medicine, biennial.

Information Industry Directory. Detroit, Gale Research Co., annual.

Nolan, Kathleen Lopez. *Gale Directory of Databases*. Detroit, Gale Research, Inc., 1995.

Roper, Fred W. and Jo Anne Boorkman. *Introduction to Reference Sources in the Health Sciences.* 3rd ed. Chicago, Medical Library Association, c1994.

The SALIS Directory: Substance Abuse Librarians and Information Specialists. 2nd ed. Berkeley, Calif., Alcohol Research Group, Medical Research Institute of San Francisco and University of California, Berkeley, 1991.

Statistics Sources. 19th ed. Detroit, Gale Research Inc., 1996.

7. JOURNAL LISTINGS

*The Serials Directory. An International Reference Book. Birmingham, Ebsco Publishing, annual (supplemented by quarterly updates).

**Ulrich's International Periodicals Directory, Now Including Irregular Serials & Annuals.* New York, R. R. Bowker Co., annual (updated between editions by *Ulrich's Quarterly*).

> See: Subject categories, such as drug abuse and alcoholism, medical sciences, pharmacy and pharmacology, psychology, public health and safety.

8. AUDIOVISUAL PROGRAMS

The Directory of Medical Video Programs. Hawthorne, N.J., Ridge Publishing Co., 1990.

**National Library of Medicine Audiovisuals Catalog.* Bethesda, Md., National Library of Medicine, 1977-1993, quarterly, with annual cumulations.

> See: *MeSH* terms as noted in Section 1 under *Index Medicus.*

Patient Education Sourcebook. 2v. Saint Louis, Mo., Health Sciences Communications Association, c1985-90.

> See: *MeSH* terms as noted in Section 1 under *Index Medicus.*

9. GUIDES TO UPCOMING MEETINGS

Scientific Meetings. San Diego, Calif., Scientific Meetings Publications, quarterly.

> See: Subject indexes.

> See: Association listing.

World Meetings: Medicine. New York, Macmillan Pub. Co., quarterly.

> See: Keyword index.

> See: Sponsor directory and index.

World Meetings: Outside United States and Canada. New York, Macmillan Pub. Co., quarterly.

> See: Keyword index.

> See: Sponsor directory and index.

World Meetings: United States and Canada. New York, Macmillan Pub. Co., quarterly.

> See: Keyword index.

> See: Sponsor directory and index.

10. PROCEEDINGS OF MEETINGS

*Directory of Published Proceedings. Series SEMT. Science/Engineering/ Medicine/Technology. White Plains, N.Y., InterDok Corp., v.3, 1967- , monthly, except July-August, with annual cumulations.

*Index to Scientific and Technical Proceedings. Philadelphia, Institute for Scientific Information, 1978- , monthly with semiannual cumulations.

11. SPECIALIZED RESEARCH CENTERS

Medical Research Centres. Harlow, Essex, Longman, biennial.

International Research Centers Directory. Detroit, Gale Research Co., annual.

Research Centers Directory. Detroit, Gale Research Co., annual (updated by *New Research Centers*).

12. SPECIAL LIBRARY COLLECTIONS

Directory of Special Libraries and Information Centers. Detroit, Gale Research Co., annual (updated by *New Special Libraries*).

Index

Page numbers followed by letter "t" designate tables; and numbers followed by "f" designate figures.